Physiotherapy Secrets
Multiple Choice Questions

Physiotherapy Secrets
Multiple Choice Questions

PP Mohanty MPT (Rehab)
Associate Professor and HOD, Physiotherapy
Swami Vivekananda National Institute of Rehabilitation
Training and Research (SVNIRTAR)
Cuttack, Orissa (India)

Monalisa Pattnaik MPT (Cardio-pulm)
Lecturer, Physiotherapy
Swami Vivekananda National Institute of Rehabilitation
Training and Research (SVNIRTAR)
Cuttack, Orissa (India)

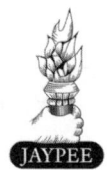

JAYPEE BROTHERS MEDICAL PUBLISHERS
The Health Sciences Publisher
New Delhi | London

Jaypee Brothers Medical Publishers (P) Ltd.

Headquarters
Jaypee Brothers Medical Publishers (P) Ltd
23/23-B, Ansari Road, Daryaganj
New Delhi 110 002, India
Phone: +91-11-23272143, +91-11-23272703
+91-11-23282021, +91-11-23245672
E-mail: jaypee@jaypeebrothers.com

Corporate Office
Jaypee Brothers Medical Publishers (P) Ltd.
4838/24, Ansari Road, Daryaganj
New Delhi 110 002, India
Phone: +91-11-43574357
Fax: +91-11-43574314
E-mail: jaypee@jaypeebrothers.com

Overseas Office
JP Medical Ltd
83 Victoria Street, London
SW1H 0HW (UK)
Phone: +44 20 3170 8910
E-mail: info@jpmedpub.com

EU GPSR Authorised Representative
Logos Europe, 9 rue Nicolas Poussin
17000, La Rochelle, France
Phone: +33 (0) 6 67 93 73 78
E-mail: Contact@logoseurope.eu

Website: www.jaypeebrothers.com
Website: www.jaypeedigital.com

© 2008, Jaypee Brothers Medical Publishers

The views and opinions expressed in this book are solely those of the original contributor(s)/author(s) and do not necessarily represent those of editor(s) and publisher of the book.

All rights reserved. No part of this publication may be reproduced, stored or transmitted in any form or by any means, electronic, mechanical, photocopying, recording or otherwise, without the prior permission in writing of the publishers.

All brand names and product names used in this book are trade names, service marks, trademarks or registered trademarks of their respective owners. The publisher is not associated with any product or vendor mentioned in this book.

Medical knowledge and practice change constantly. This book is designed to provide accurate, authoritative information about the subject matter in question. However, readers are advised to check the most current information available on procedures included and check information from the manufacturer of each product to be administered, to verify the recommended dose, formula, method and duration of administration, adverse effects and contraindications. It is the responsibility of the practitioner to take all appropriate safety precautions. Neither the publisher nor the author(s)/editor(s) assume any liability for any injury and/or damage to persons or property arising from or related to use of material in this book.

This book is sold on the understanding that the publisher is not engaged in providing professional medical services. If such advice or services are required, the services of a competent medical professional should be sought.

Every effort has been made where necessary to contact holders of copyright to obtain permission to reproduce copyright material. If any have been inadvertently overlooked, the publisher will be pleased to make the necessary arrangements at the first opportunity.

Inquiries for bulk sales may be solicited at: jaypee@jaypeebrothers.com

Physiotherapy Secrets

First Edition : 2008
   Reprint : 2025

ISBN: 978-81-8448-355-0

Printed in India at Sterling Graphics Pvt. Ltd.

To
*Baba, without your love we would
not have been able to achieve our goal.*
Lulu
Luna

Preface

This book is intended primarily for bachelor of physiotherapy students who prepare for their university examinations or for postgraduate entrance examinations. We think that it will also be useful for physiotherapists attending the licensing examination of other countries.

We have attempted to cover different areas of physical therapy.

We have used many generally accepted abbreviations.

Despite our best efforts some errors might have crept in. In case of any query please write to us.

We like to thank all those who have helped us.

PP Mohanty
Monalisa Pattnaik

Contents

1. Exercise Therapy *1*
2. Electrotherapy *28*
3. Physiotherapy in Orthopaedic Conditions *57*
4. Physiotherapy in Neurological Conditions *103*
5. Physiotherapy in Cardiopulmonary
   Conditions *139*
6. Biomechanics *164*
7. Rehabilitation *182*
8. Physiotherapy in Surgical Conditions..................... *193*
9. Alternative Medicine *201*
10. Biostatistics *207*

CHAPTER 1

Exercise Therapy

1. The effect of two non-linear force systems acting at a common point can be determined by finding out their resultant, which can be determined by____
   a. Simple arithmetic addition   b. Law of triangle
   c. Law of parallelogram d. Cosine law
2. 40 Kg traction force is applied to the part at an angle of 30 degrees. What will be the effective distractive force at the joint?
   a. 30kg   b. 35kg
   c. 40 kg   d. 45 kg
3. Friction is the resistive force offered by the surface, when one surface moves over the other, which is directly proportional to____.
   a. The area of the surface in contact
   b. Nature of the surface
   c. Weight of the moving object
   d. All of the above
4. Pulleys are used to _____.
   a. Make the work easy
   b. Alter the direction of motion
   c. Gain mechanical efficiency
   d. All the above
5. In a pulley maximum resistance force is produced when the angle of pulley is_____.
   a. In line with the moving bone

b. 90⁰ to the moving bone
   c. 60⁰ with moving bone
   d. 45⁰ with the moving bone
6. _____ order lever is the lever of speed.
   a. 1st				b. 2nd
   c. 3rd				d. All
7. Knee flexion in prone lying is an example of_____.
   a. 1st order lever		b. 2nd order lever
   c. 3rd order lever		d. 4th order lever
8. 2nd order lever is the lever of_____.
   a. Stability			b. Instability
   c. Speed			d. Efficiency
9. Standing on toes is an example of _____ order lever.
   a. 1st				b. 2nd
   c. 3rd				d. 4th
10. In our body more numbers of _____ order levers are present
    a. 1st				b. 2nd
    c. 3rd				d. 4th
11. ___ order lever is the lever of power.
    a. 1st				b. 2nd
    c. 3rd				d. All
12. Nodding movement of head is the example of _____ order lever.
    a. 1st				b. 2nd
    c. 3rd				d. 4th
13. Elbow flexion in mid-prone position is done by brachioradialis muscle; lifting 10 kg dumb-bell converts it from _____.
    a. 1st to 2nd order lever	b. 2nd to 3rd order lever
    c. 3rd to 4th order lever	d. 3rd to 1st order lever all
14. The degrees of freedom of the MCPJ of fingers is____.
    a. 1				b. 2
    c. 3				d. 4
15. Ankle DF/PF takes place _____.
    a. Saggital plane and frontal axis
    b. Frontal plane and saggital axis
    c. Transverse plane and vertical axis
    d. Coronal plane and horizontal axis

16. The characteristics of any starting position _____.
    a. Stable
    b. Comfortable
    c. Provide room for full range of motion
    d. All of the above
17. Active fixation can be achieved by _____.
    a. Co-contraction of muscles
    b. Straps
    c. Manual pressure
    d. Non of the above
18. In normal standing, line of gravity passes_____the knee joint.
    a. In front of   b. Behind
    c. Through   d. Lateral to
19. Pronation and supination take place on _____.
    a. Sagittal plane and frontal axis
    b. Frontal plane and sagittal axis
    c. Transverse plane and vertical axis
    d. Coronal plane and horizontal axis
20. Mechanically the assistance/ resistance are most effective when it acts at ___.
    a. Acute angle   b. Obtuse angle
    c. Perpendicular   d. Zero degree
21. Muscle is most efficient in_____ range.
    a. Outer   b. Outer part of middle
    c. Inner part of middle d. Inner
22. Forearm pronation range of motion is limited due to _____.
    a. Bony contact
    b. Soft tissue approximation
    c. Soft tissue tension
    d. Tension of ligament
23. Relaxed passive movement is useful for_____.
    a. Muscle strengthening
    b. Improving joint range of motion
    c. Remembrance of pattern of movement
    d. Improving co-ordination

24. Stretching is the _____.
    a. Slow and sustained forced passive movement
    b. Sudden but controlled forced passive movement
    c. Relaxed passive movement
    d. Manipulation
25. Anterior pelvic tilt is produced by _____.
    a. Hip extensors and abdominals
    b. hip flexors and lumbar extensors
    c. Hip adductors and trunk side flexors
    d. Non of the above
26. Natural speed for every active exercise varies from individual to individual and in the same individual from time to time. Choose the correct answer regarding the speed of movement.
    a. Concentric work at increased or decreased speed requires greater muscular effort
    b. Muscle contraction at natural speed is most efficient
    c. Eccentric work at increased speed is easy
    d. All of the above
27. Muscles are most often used in the middle range during activities of daily livings, so most efficient within this range.
    a. Exercise in outer range is used for muscle re-education
    b. Exercise in middle range is used for muscle tone and power
    c. Exercise in inner range is used for training stabilization
    d. All of the above
28. Finger walking on the wall to touch a mark is an example of _____ exercise.
    a. Passive
    b. Subjective free
    c. Objective free
    d. Assisted
29. In which of the PRE the load remains constant during the training session_____.
    a. Delorme   b. Watkin
    c. Zinovief   d. McQueen

30. In Delorme's PRE the progression of 10 RM is made once in _____.
    a. Daily   b. Every week
    c. Every fortnight   d. Every month
31. Low resistance high repetition exercise is used to improve muscle_____.
    a. Strength   b. Endurance
    c. Volume   d. Co-ordination
32. Example of soft tissue approximation limiting joint range of motion is____.
    a. Forearm supination
    b. Hip flexion with knee extension
    c. Ankle dorsiflexion with knee flexion
    d. Elbow flexion
33. Example of passive insufficiency is _____.
    a. Hip flexion with knee extension
    b. Fingers flexion with wrist extension
    c. Ankle dorsiflexion with knee flexion
    d. Shoulder external rotation with abduction
34. Limitation of finger abduction is due to tension of _____.
    a. Skin   b. Muscles
    c. Ligament   d. Bone
35. End feel of _____ is bony.
    a. Knee extension
    b. Elbow extension
    c. Ankle dorsiflexion
    d. Forearm supination
36. Forced passive movement is contraindicated for _____ joint.
    a. Hip   b. Knee
    c. Elbow   d. Spine
37. Joint mobilization is contraindicated in _____.
    a. Soft tissue tightness
    b. Joint stiffness
    c. Loose body inside the joint
    d. Bursitis
38. Glenohumeral anterior glide can improve
    a. Extension range
    b. Flexion range

    c. Extension and external rotation
    d. Flexion and internal rotation range
39. Kaltenborn has described _____ grades
    a. 4   b. 3
    c. 5   d. None of the above.
40. Ankle traction can improve _____ range of motion.
    a. Plantar flexion   b. Dorsi flexion
    c. Inversion   d. Eversion
41. Leathery end feel is characteristic of _____.
    a. Soft tissue tightness
    b. Capsular tightness
    c. Bony obstruction
    d. Internal derangement
42. The end feel of loose body inside the joint is _____.
    a. Elastic   b. Hard
    c. Leathery   d. Springy rebound
43. The fixed point in axial suspension is _____.
    a. Vertically above the axis of the joint
    b. Vertically above the cg of the part
    c. Sideways to the anatomical axis of the joint
    d. Sideways to the CG of the part
44. Pendular suspension is used to improve the JROM by shifting the fixed point of the axial suspension____
    a. Towards the direction of motion
    b. Opposite to the direction of motion
    c. Upward
    d. Downward
45. In axial suspension the part rests in ____ position.
    a. Neutral
    b. Away from neutral
    c. Above the supporting surface
    d. Flexion
46. Movement in pendular suspension takes place in _____ plane.
    a. Horizontal   b. Inclined plane
    c. Sagittal   d. Frontal
47. Double pulley rope is used to support heavy body part, it becomes _____.
    a. Difficult to elevate the part by lifting the wooden cleat up

b. Possible to do 3-D movements
   c. Easy to elevate the part by pulling the wooden cleat down
   d. None of the above
48. Vertical suspension is used for _____.
   a. Relaxation
   b. Strengthening
   c. Stretching
   d. Proximal fixation
49. Pulley rope in suspension therapy is used to _____.
   a. Elevate the part from the supporting surface
   b. Permits 3d pattern of movements
   c. Allow frictionless to and fro movements
   d. All of the above
50. Choose the correct statement
   a. Physiological cost of concentric muscle work is greater than eccentric
   b. Physiological cost of static muscle work is greater than concentric
   c. Physiological cost of eccentric muscle work is greater than concentric
   d. Physiological cost of isometric muscle work is greater than eccentric
51. Which of the following statements is true regarding muscle strengthening?
   a. Increase and decrease in speed of movement is a progression of concentric work
   b. Increase in speed of movement is a progression of eccentric work
   c. Decrease in speed of movement is a progression of static work
   d. All of the above
52. Frenkel's exercises are devised to improve co-ordination by use of sight, sound and touch in case of ataxia due to_____.
   a. Cerebellar lesion
   b. Loss of kinesthetic sensation
   c. Spastic paralysis
   d. Flaccid paralysis

53. Progression of Frenkel's exercise is made by alteration of ____.
    a. Speed- Quick to slow
    b. Range- wider to smaller
    c. Complexity of exercises
    d. All of the above
54. For the recovering muscles _____.
    a. Concentric exercises are given before eccentric
    b. Eccentric exercises are given before concentric
    c. Concentric and eccentric exercises are given together
    d. Eccentric exercises are given before static
55. PNF was developed by_____.
    a. Kabat and Knott
    b. Knot and Voss
    c. Car and Shepherd
    d. Dardiner and Hollis
56. Which of the following PNF techniques is used in Cerebellar ataxia?
    a. Repeated contraction
    b. Hold and relax
    c. Rhythmic initiation
    d. Rhythmic stabilization
57. Rhythmic Initiation technique is used for _____.
    a. Tightness
    b. Flaccid paralysis
    c. Cerebellar ataxia
    d. Parkinsonism
58. Groove in PNF refers to_____.
    a. Maximum resistacce
    b. Diagnonal pattern of movement
    c. Repeatition
    d. Proprioceptive stimuli
59. In PNF elbow flexion is a component of _____.
    a. Flexion- abduction – external rotation
    b. Flexion- adduction – external rotation
    c. Extension- abduction – internal rotation
    d. All of the above

60. In PNF knee flexion is a component of _____.
    a. Flexion- abduction – external rotation
    b. Flexion- adduction – external rotation
    c. Extension- adduction – internal rotation
    d. Extension- abduction – external rotation
61. Which is not true for rhythmic stabilization?
    a. It develops co-contraction
    b. Manual resistance applied alternately to opposite side only in closed kinematic chain position
    c. It develops stability
    d. There should not be any relaxation phase between contraction.
62. Choose the correct progression of ambulation by a pair of auxiliary crutches_____.
    a. 2 point, 3 point , 4 point
    b. 4 point, 3 point, 2 point
    c. 3 point, 4 point, 2 point
    d. 2 point, 4 point, 3 point
63. The correct sequence of stair climbing with a pair of axillary crutches is_____.
    a. Crutches, affected leg, sound leg
    b. Affected leg, sound leg, crutches
    c. Sound leg , affected leg, crutches
    d. Crutches, , sound leg, affected leg
64. Elbow crutches are indicated for the persons with _____.
    a. Strong upper extremities and strong trunk
    b. Strong upper extremities and weak trunk
    c. Weak upper extremities and strong trunk
    d. Weak upper extremities and weak trunk
65. Gutter crutches are indicated for the persons with _____.
    a. Strong upper extremities and strong trunk
    b. Strong upper extremities and weak trunk
    c. Strong upper extremities but problems in FA/wrist and hand and strong trunk
    d. Strong upper extremities but problems in FA/wrist and hand and weak trunk

66. Persons with unilateral hip problem leans to the affected side and advised to use a walking stick. On which side he should use the stick?
    a. Affected side
    b. Sound side
    c. Either side
    d. Single stick is not useful
67. The measurement for axillary crutches is taken from _____.
    a. Anterior axillary fold to 20 cm forward and lateral to little toe
    b. Tip of the axilla to 20 cm forward and lateral to little toe
    c. Anterior axillary fold to tip of medial malleolus
    d. All of the above
68. While descending the stairs, the therapist must stand_____.
    a. Behind the patient
    b. Behind the patient towards the weaker side
    c. In front of the patient
    d. In front of the patient towards the weaker side
69. Trendelenburg's sign is said to be positive, when_____.
    a. Sound side pelvis drop down, while standing on affected side
    b. Affected side pelvis drop down, while standing on sound side
    c. Sound side pelvis elevated, while standing on affected side
    d. None of the above
70. In Thomas test position limitation of hip adduction range indicates shortening of __.
    a. TFL
    b. ITB
    c. Iliopsoas
    d. Rectus femoris
71. In Thomas test position limitation of hip internal rotation range indicates shortening of _____.
    a. TFL
    b. ITB
    c. Iliopsoas
    d. Rectus femoris

72. Sterncledomastoid tightness is characterized by _____ deformity.
    a. Neck side flexion towards the affected side with rotation to opposite side
    b. Neck side flexion towards the sound side with rotation to affected side
    c. Neck side flexion and rotation towards the affected side
    d. Neck side flexion and rotation towards the sound side
73. Ober's test is done to detect shortening of _____.
    a. Iliopsoas   b. IT band
    c. hamstrings   d. Gastro-soleus
74. Hip abductors at grade 3 is tested in inside lying on the sound side. For gluteus minimus hip abduction is done _____.
    a. In neutral position
    b. In flexion
    c. In extension
    d. In external rotation
75. To test Quadriceps for grade 2, the subject should lay _____.
    a. On affected side   b. On sound
    c. In supine   d. In prone
76. During elbow flexion in sitting, Triceps _____.
    a. Works concentrically
    b. Works eccentrically
    c. Works statically
    d. Does not work
77. Leg lowering from extended knee position, Quadriceps works _____.
    a. Concentrically
    b. Eccentrically
    c. Statically
    d. Isokinetically
78. Leg lowering against resistance from extended knee position, _____.
    a. Quadriceps works concentrically
    b. Quadriceps works eccentrically

c. Hamstrings works concentrically
d. Hamstrings works eccentrically

79. What should be the temperature of water in hydrotherapy unit?
    a. 27 C – 35 C
    b. 22 C – 42 C
    c. 32 C – 35 C
    d. None of the above

80. In hydrotherapy the factor/factors which can have an effect on heart rate is/are_____.
    a. Temperature of water
    b. Hydrostatic pressure of water
    c. Both a and b
    d. Buoyancy of water

81. The upward movement inside the water is easy. The movement is assisted by ____.
    a. Gravity
    b. Buoyancy
    c. Hydrostatic pressure
    d. Water current

82. Which of the following properties of water helps a patient with lower extremity muscles weakness to stand inside hydrotherapy pool, which otherwise can not stand?
    a. Buoyancy
    b. Temperature of water
    c. Hydrostatic pressure
    d. Specific gravity

83. The cross infection in hydrotherapy can be checked by_____.
    a. Boiling the water
    b. Washing the client before entering into the pool
    c. Controlling the environmental temperature, humidity etc.
    d. Chlorinating the water

84. Movement on the surface of the water is _____.
    a. Assisted buoyancy
    b. Free
    c. Supported by hydrostatic pressure
    d. Resisted by the displaced water

85. The dangers of hydrotherapy is_____.
    a. Slippage and fall   b. Drowning
    c. Infection   d. All of the above
86. The danger of prolonged hydrotherapy is _____.
    a. Fatigue
    b. Water and electrolyte loss
    c. Rise in body temperature
    d. All the above
87. The contraindication of hydrotherapy is_____.
    a. Convulsions
    b. Respiratory diseases
    c. Incontinence of bowel and bladder
    d. All the above
88. Which of the following properties of water helps a patient with lower extremity muscles weakness to stand in side hydrotherapy pool, which otherwise can not stand?
    a. Buoyancy
    b. Temperature of water
    c. Hydrostatic pressure
    d. Specific gravity
89. For group therapy, maximum number of patients in group is about _____.
    a. 4-6   b. 6-8
    c. 8-10   d. More than 10
90. The advantages of group therapy _____.
    a. Time saving for therapist
    b. Builds up confidence in patients
    c. Maximizes patient's effort and develop competition among the patients
    d. All the above
91. Mitchell technique of relaxation is based on the principle of _____.
    a. Reciprocal innervations
    b. Autogenic inhibition
    c. Cue controlled relaxation
    d. Released only
92. Valsalva Maneuver should be avoided for_____.
    a. Patients with hypertension
    b. Geriatric patients

c. Patients who have undergone abdominal surgery
d. All of the above

93. Progressive resistance exercises improve the muscle power in every individual_____.
    a. True
    b. false
    c. Not always

94. Delayed onset muscle soreness peaks at_____.
    a. 1 – 2 days.
    b. 2 – 3 days.
    c. 1 week
    d. None of the above

95. DOMS can be prevented by_____.
    a. Adding warm up and cool down period to the exercise protocol
    b. By a gradually progressive exercise programme
    c. Achieving sretchability in the exercising muscle prior to the exercise programme
    d. All of the above

96. If stair climbing has to be improved which exercises should be done?
    a. Closed chain concentric
    b. Closed chain concentric and eccentric
    c. Closed and open chain concentric and eccentric
    d. Open chain concentric exercises.

97. To improve function which exercise programme is preferable?
    a. Closed chain concentric
    b. Open chain concentric
    c. Plyometric
    d. Closed chain concentric and eccentric

98. Which is not true for isokinetic exercise?
    a. Exercise speed can vary from very low to very high speed
    b. Strength gain occurs at training speed
    c. Patient need to control the momentum.
    d. It improves muscle endurance

99. Which is the most important variable to improve muscle force generation capacity?
    a. Load
    b. Duration
    c. Sets
    d. Frequency

100. The minimum duration of exercise programme to improve strength should be at least_____.
    a. 3 weeks
    b. 6 weeks
    c. 10 weeks
    d. 12 weeks
101. What should be the progression of exercise protocol following musculoskeletal injury?
    a. Isometric – eccentric – concentric
    b. Isometric – concentric – concentric and eccentric
    c. Concentric – eccentric – concentric and eccentric
    d. Isometric - concentric – eccentric
102. Oxford technique is opposite of_____.
    a. Dapre
    b. Delorme
    c. Mcqueen
    d. None of the above
103. In slow stretching_____.
    a. GTO fires
    b. Muscle spindle fires
    c. Monosynaptic stretch reflex initiated
    d. None of the above
104. Tightness is same as_____.
    a. Scar tissue adhesion
    b. Adaptive shortening
    c. Transient contracture
    d. Contracture.
105. When there is permanent deformation with a load of low magnitude and long duration in the elastic range it is known as_____.
    a. Fatigue failure
    b. Reaching elastic limit
    c. Creep
    d. Ultimate strength.
106. For most of our functional activities we use_____.
    a. Toe region of collagen fibres
    b. Elastic portion of collagen fibre
    c. Plastic range
    d. None of the above
107. Which is the best method for stretching tight structures?
    a. Manual stretch
    b. Prolonged cyclic
    c. Prolonged sustained stretching
    d. Ballistic stretching

108. In any exercise programme for 1 MET increase of exercise level systolic blood pressure rises by_____.
    a. 5 – 7 mmHg
    b. 7 – 10 mmHg
    c. 10 – 12 mmHg
    d. 12 – 15 mmHg
109. Active inhibition techniques are not effective for_____.
    a. Muscle Weakness
    b. Spasticity
    c. Paralysis form neuromuscular dysfunction
    d. All of the above
110. Volume of training refers to_____.
    a. Intensity multiplied by duration
    b. Total number of sets
    c. Sets multiplied by resistance
    d. None of the above
111. Usually more than _____ sets cause musculoskeltal injury
    a. 2 set
    b. 3 set
    c. 5 set
    d. 10 set
112. In DAPRE the base repetition maximum is_____.
    a. 10 RM
    b. 1 RM
    c. 6 RM
    d. 3 RM
113. To avoid muscle strain which is important among the following?
    a. Adequate strength
    b. Adequate extensibility
    c. Adequate resistance to fatigue
    d. All of the above
114. Which is not true in case of muscle strengthening.
    a. Cross sectional area of the muscle increase
    b. Number of muscle fibre increase
    c. Mitochondrial density increases
    d. Energy sources for muscle activity increases
115. Which is the important factor to gain bone density?
    a. Resistance training
    b. Weight bearing aerobic conditioning
    c. Weight bearing resistance training
    d. Non-weight bearing aerobic training

116. Which is not an effect of strengthening on CVS?
    a. Increased heart rate
    b. Decreased systolic BP
    c. Increased cardiac output
    d. Decreased cholesterol
117. Which is not true for endurance training?
    a. Increased use of fatty acid
    b. Increase used of glycogen
    c. Slowing accumulation of lactic acid in the working muscle
    d. None of the above
118. ACSM classifies for muscle strengthening programme, a person with 6 months of consistent resistance training experience as_____.
    a. Novice   b. Intermediate
    c. Advanced   d. Elite
119. What is the % gain expected from untrained individual?
    a. Upto 10 %   b. Upto 20 %
    c. Upto 40%   d. Upto 60 %
120. How much gain in strength is expected from elite individual?
    a. 2 %   b. 5 %
    c. 10%   d. 15 %
121. What is the optimal time of hold necessary for isometric contractions?
    a. 6 seconds   b. 10 seconds
    c. 12 seconds   d. 12 seconds
122. The advantage of isometric contraction could be because it_____.
    a. Helps for re – education
    b. Helps gaining muscle strength
    c. Prepares for dynamic exercise
    d. All of the above
123. Hypertensive can do isometrics with a hold period of____.
    a. < 1 sec   b. < 2 sec
    c. < 3 sec   d. < 5 sec

124. The cam system used in a weight machine provides_____.
    a. Constant resistance
    b. Less resistance when patient is exhausted
    c. Less resistance at he beginning and end of ROM
    d. Gives resistance intermittently
125. Which is not an advantage of weight machine?
    a. There is effective stabilization
    b. There is gain in proprioception and balance
    c. They are time efficient
    d. The equipment is time efficient
126. If balance is the rehabilitation goal which exercise programme is preferred?
    a. Weight machine
    b. Free machine
    c. Both have similar advantage for balance
    d. Pulley or cam machine
127. Hopping, skipping, jumping are form of_____.
    a. Eccentric exercise
    b. Plyometrics
    c. Concentric followed by eccentric
    d. None of the above
128. The distinction of impact activities and plyometrics is its_____.
    a. Eccentric phase
    b. For production
    c. Amortization phase
    d. Velocity of phases
129. Which is more functional speed in isokinetic training?
    a. High   b. Intermediate
    c. Low   d. Low followed by high
130. Ballistic stretching is helpful for _____.
    a. Musculoskeletal patients
    b. Neurological patients
    c. Athletes
    d. All of the above.
131. If stretching is done upto 5 times with duration of stretch 30 sec. the length gain may last upto _____.
    a. 5 minutes   b. 10 minutes
    c. ½ hour   d. 1 hour.

132. If 6 week stretching Programme is given, we expect the retention of gain up to _____.
    a. 1 month
    b. 2 months
    c. 3 months
    d. 6 months.
133. For elderly individual the duration of stretch should be _____.
    a. Same as younger individuals
    b. More than young people
    c. Less than young people
    d. Should not be given stretching.
134. Double support phase present at the _____ phase of gait cycle.
    a. Beginning of stance
    b. End of stance
    c. Beginning and end of stance
    d. Mid stance
135. The CG displaced to the highest level during _____ phase of gait cycle
    a. Foot flat
    b. Mid stance
    c. Double support
    d. Mid Swing
136. Horizontal displacement of CG during normal human locomotion is about _____.
    a. 2 cm
    b. 5 cm
    c. 7 cm
    d. 10 cm
137. Cadence is the number of steps per minute, which is equal to _____ in normal human locomotion.
    a. 70 – 90
    b. 90 – 110
    c. 90 – 130
    d. 70 – 130
138. During normal human locomotion knee movement is co-ordinated with ankle movement to minimize the upward displacement of CG. The relationship between knee and ankle movements are_____.
    a. Knee flexion occurs with ankle dorsiflexion
    b. Knee extension occurs with ankle plantarflexion
    c. Knee flexion occurs with ankle plantarflexion
    d. None of the above

139. At heel strike phase of gait cycle line of gravity passes behind the ankle joint creating plantar flexion moment, so _____.
   a. Dorsiflexors act eccentrically
   b. Dorsiflexors act concentrically
   c. Plantarflexors act eccentrically
   d. Plantarflexors act concentrically
140. At midstance phase of gait cycle line of gravity passes in front of the hip joint creating flexion moment. Weakness of Gluteus maximus gives rise to _____ gait.
   a. Hand to thigh gait
   b. Anterior trunk bending
   c. Posterior lurching
   d. Hip hiking
141. Stiff knee gait is characterized by _____.
   a. Lurching
   b. Hand to knee
   c. Hip hiking
   d. Steppage gait
142. Foot supination takes place during _____ phase of gait cycle.
   a. Heel strike to foot flat
   b. Foot flat to mid stance
   c. Mid stance to heel up
   d. Heel up to toe up
143. _____ muscle is known as decelerator in normal human locomotion.
   a. Iliopsoas
   b. Gastrosoleus
   c. Hamstring
   d. Quadriceps
144. Running is distinguished from walking by _____.
   a. Cadence more than 130/min.
   b. Absence of double support phase
   c. All of the above
145. Person with hip abductors weakness walks with lateral trunk bending towards the affected side during the stance phase, which___.
   a. Improves the efficacy of hip abductors
   b. Shifts the weight line towards the involved side
   c. Gives rise to apparent weight loss
   d. Provides momentum

146. Person with Quadriceps weakness walks with equines gait, correction of which
    a. Will loose the independent ambulation
    b. Improves the cosmesis and function
    c. Strengthen the Quadriceps
    d. None of the above
147. _____ manipulation is used to obtain sensory stimulation.
    a. Stroking   b. Effleurage
    c. Kneading   d. Friction
148. Which of the following is not a tapotement technique?
    a. Clapping   b. Beating
    c. Pounding   d. Petrissage
149. The movement required for hacking manipulation is_____.
    a. Forearm supination - pronation
    b. Wrist flexion – extension
    c. Elbow flexion – extension
    d. All of the above
150. A pillow is placed under the abdomen in prone lying position for the massage of the back to ____.
    a. Flatten the back
    b. Raise the pelvis to facilitate drainage
    c. Relieve pressure over the breasts in case of female
    d. All of the above
151. The benefits of correct Therapist's position ___.
    a. Stress on therapist's back is reduced
    b. Little energy expenditure as body weight is used
    c. Direction, pressure and rhythm of movements are easily controlled
    d. All of the above
152. For the effective stretching of the hip flexors _____.
    a. Lay in prone
    b. In prone position at the edge of the bed, hold the sound hip in full flexion out of the bed
    c. In supine lying position at the edge of the bed, hold the sound hip in full flexion and hold the involved side foot to pull the thigh downward out of the bed
    d. All of the above

153. Quadriceps in grade 3 usually tested in high sitting position, which does not allow full range of motion. More suitable position is _____.
    a. Supine lying
    b. Supine lying with the thigh fixed at about 90 of flexion
    c. Sit lying
    d. Standing
154. Trick movement for weak quadriceps is _____.
    a. Hip extension by Gluteus maximus, which extends the knee through ITB
    b. Hip flexion by TFL, which extends the knee through ITB
    c. Both a and b
    d. None of the above
155. Hip flexors for grade 3 should be tested in standing; but the person who cannot stand; it is tested in high sitting position, which does not allow full range of motion. More suitable position is _____.
    a. Supine lying
    b. Supine lying with the thigh fixed at about 90 of flexion
    c. Sit lying
    d. None of the above
156. Hamstrings in grade 3 usually tested in prone lying position, which allows only 90 of knee flexion against gravity. To achieve full knee flexion against gravity standing position is selected; but the person who cannot stand, it can be tested in _____.
    a. Trunk prone lying
    b. Prone kneeling
    c. Hanging
    d. None of the above
157. To test for grade 4 and 5, check the maximum resistance on the sound side and then apply_____ on the involved side and compare the both.
    a. Minimum resistance
    b. Same resistance
    c. Maximum possible resistance, which one can overcome
    d. None of the above

158. Simple objective method of muscle evaluation can be done by _____.
    a. Manual muscle testing
    b. 1 repetition maximum
    c. Isokinetic device
    d. Dynamometer
159. Trunk rotation to right side is produced by _____.
    a. Internal oblique of right side and external rotation of left
    b. Both internal oblique and external rotation of right side
    c. Internal oblique of left side and external rotation of right
    d. Both internal oblique and external rotation of left side
160. For goniometry _____ is done first.
    a. Align the fixed arm with the proximal segment
    b. Align the movable arm with the distal segment
    c. Align the axis over the anatomical axis of the joint
    d. None of the above
161. Range of glenohumeral abduction is about _____.
    a. 180   b. 160
    c. 100-110   d. 90
162. Carpometacarpal joint of thumb has got _____ degrees of freedom
    a. 1   b. 2
    c. 3   d. 4
163. _____ joint has got one degree of freedom
    a. Ankle
    b. Elbow
    c. Interphalangeal
    d. All of the above
164. The factor limiting knee joint range of motion is _____.
    a. Bony contact
    b. Tension of the skin
    c. Tension of the posterior capsule
    d. Tension of hamstrings

165. The factor limiting glenohumeral abduction joint range of motion is _____.
    a. Contact between greater tuberosity and acromion
    b. Unavailability of articular surface over the head of the humerus
    c. Tension of the joint capsule
    d. All of the above
166. In case of pain and progressive limitation of elbow joint range of motion, _____ is recommended.
    a. Rest
    b. Mobilization
    c. Manipulation
    d. None of the above
167. During inspiration the anteroposterior diameter of thoracic cage increases by _____.
    a. Downward excursion of diaphragm
    b. Bucket handle movements of lower ribs
    c. Pump handle movements of upper ribs
    d. All of the above
168. Respiratory excursion is highest in _____.
    a. Supine lying
    b. Sitting
    c. Standing
    d. Kneel standing
169. In breath control, the subject is instructed to breathe at _____.
    a. Normal tidal volume
    b. Increased tidal volume
    c. Decreased tidal volume
    d. According to Therapist's verbal command
170. The principle of Frenkel's co-ordination exercises is/are _____.
    a. Precision   b. Attention
    c. Repetition   d. All of the above
171. Progression of Frenkel's co-ordination exercises is made by _____.
    a. Alteration speed of movements i.e. slow and fast
    b. Alteration range of motion i.e. wider to small

c. Adding more complex movements i.e. hip movement is followed by hip and knee movements
d. Changing non-weight bearing to weight bearing
e. All of the above
172. Engram formation for co-ordination needs _____ repetition of precise movements.
    a. 100 million   b. 200 million
    c. 300 million   d. 400 million
173. Good posture _____.
    a. Saves energy
    b. Looks aesthetically good
    c. Prevents musculoskeletal complications
    d. All of the above
174. Poor posture _____.
    a. Energy consuming, so gives rise to early fatigue
    b. Looks aesthetically ugly
    c. Gives rise to painful musculoskeletal problems
    d. All of the above
175. Elbow joint is the site of the common cause of the myositis ossificans. Which muscle is he most commonly involved?
    a. Biceps brachi
    b. Brachioradialis
    c. Triceps
    d. Brachialis
176. Push up is an example of _____.
    a. Close kinetic chain exercise
    b. Active free weight bearing exercise
    c. Both a and b
    d. Resisted exercise.
177. Eccentric muscle work refers to _____.
    a. Lengthening and narrowing of muscle
    b. Antagonistic group of muscles work to control the movement
    c. Physiological cost is less, consume less oxygen; so efficient
    d. All of the above
178. Plyometric training is given for the young active individuals during the late phase of rehabilitation; which refers to _____.

a. Stretch-shortening drill
   b. Multiangle resisted training
   c. Isokinetic training
   d. Concentric-eccentric exercise
179. Effects of traction depend on _____.
   a. Magnitude of tractive force and line of pull
   b. Duration of application
   c. Position of patient
   d. Nature of the surface and state of rest or motion
   e. All of the above
180. For the traction to be effective, the force must exceed the frictional resistance encountered by the body part. For lumbar traction the force should be _____.
   a. More than 1/10 of body weight
   b. More than 1/4 of body weight
   c. More than 1/3 of body weight
   d. More than 1/2 of body weight
181. Traction for the upper cervical spine problem should be given with the neck in _____ position.
   a. Neutral
   b. Slight extension
   c. Slight flexion
   d. 24 of flexion

ANSWER SHEET EXERCISE THERAPY

1. c	2. b	3. d	4. d	5. b
6. c	7. c	8. d	9. c	10. c
11. b	12. a	13. b	14. b	15. a
16. d	17. a	18. a	19. c	20. c
21. b	22. b	23. c	24. a	25. b
26. d	27. d	28. b	29. d	30. b
31. b	32. d	33. a	34. a	35. b
36. c	37. c	38. c	39. b	40. a
41. b	42. d	43. a	44. a	45. a
46. b	47. c	48. d	49. d	50. a
51. a	52. b	53. d	54. b	55. a
56. d	57. d	58. b	59. d	60. b
61. b	62. c	63. c	64. a	65. c
66. b	67. a	68. d	69. a	70. a

71. c	72. a	73. b	74. a	75. b
76. d	77. b	78. c	79. a	80. c
81. b	82. c	83. d	84. d	85. d
86. d	87. d	88. c	89. b	90. d
91. a	92. d	93. c	94. a	95. d
96. b	97. d	98. c	99. a	100. b
101. a	102. b	103. a	104. c	105. c
106. a	107. b	108. b	109. d	110. c
111. b	112. c	113. d	114. c	115. c
116. a	117. b	118. b	119. c	120. a
121. a	122. d	123. b	124. c	125. b
126. b	127. b	128. c	129. a	130. c
131. a	132. a	133. b	134. c	135. b
136. b	137. d	138. c	139. a	140. c
141. c	142. d	143. c	144. c	145. b
146. a	147. a	148. d	149. a	150. d
151. d	152. b	153. b	154. c	155. c
156. a	157. c	158. b	159. a	160. c
161. c	162. c	163. d	164. c	165. d
166. a	167. c	168. a	169. a	170. d
171. e	172. c	173. d	174. d	175. d
176. c	177. d	178. a	179. e	180. c
181. b				

# CHAPTER 2

Electrotherapy

1. What is the international color code of the active, neutral and earthed wires?
   a. Red/brown is active, black/blue is neutral and yellow/green is earthed
   b. Black/blue is active, red/brown is neutral and yellow/green is earthed
   c. Red/brown is active, yellow/green is neutral and red/brown is earthed
   d. Yellow/green is active, black/blue is neutral and red/brown is earthed
2. Which of the following factor will cause electric shock?
   a. Fault such that an exposed part of the apparatus becomes live
   b. A person makes contact with the live part
   c. The person is earthed
   d. All of the above
3. Which of the following will prevent electric shock?
   a. Use of isolated transformer, so that the current applied to the patient become earth free
   b. Incorporation of a high sensitivity core-balanced relay device/apparatus should have its own fuse
   c. The patient and apparatus should be kept distant from earthed objects e.g. metal furniture, water pipelines etc.
   d. All of the above

4. Which of the following is/are the effects of electric shock?
   a. Ventricular fibrillation
   b. Burn
   c. Muscle rupture, avulsion fracture or paralysis
   d. All of the above
5. Which of the following factor/s determines effects of electric shock?
   a. Types of current, AC is more dangerous than DC
   b. Duration of current exposure and intensity
   c. Path of current through the body
   d. All of the above
6. What are the resistances of the dry and wet skin?
   a. 10,000 – 60,000 ohm and 5,000 ohm respectively
   b. 100,000 – 600,000 ohm and 1,000 ohm respectively
   c. 10,000 – 60,000 ohm and 10,000 ohm respectively
   d. 10, 00,000 – 60, 00,000 ohm and 10,000 ohms respectively
7. The skin resistance can be reduced before applying electrical stimulation _____.
   a. Washing the skin by soap and warm water and cleaning by applying spirit or alcohol
   b. Massage the part in elevation if edema is present
   c. Soak the part with normal saline
   d. All of the above
8. Sequence of operation of electrotherapy equipments is_____.
   a. M-mains and machine on, C-clock on, P-power on
   b. P-power on, M-mains and machine on, C-clock on
   c. C-clock on, P-power on, M-mains and machine on
   d. M-mains and machine on, P-power on, C-clock on
9. Burn in electrotherapy occurs due to___.
   a. Overdose
   b. Inability to dissipate heat due to peripheral vascular disease
   c. Loss of sensation
   d. All of the above
10. Exacerbation of symptoms of symptoms following electrotherapy occurs due to___.
    a. Acute inflammation/infection

b. Area of increased fluid tension e.g. edema, effusion
   c. Haemmorrhagic conditions
   d. All of the above
11. Electrical activity in the cells of the body can be described as_____.
   a. Conduction current
   b. Convection current
   c. Both conduction and convection
   d. Radiation
12. Electrical activity of body is lower than the electrical circuits because_____.
   a. It is dependent on movement of ions
   b. Pathways are shorter
   c. The mass of ion is smaller
   d. All of the above
13. Negativity of resting membrane potential is due to _____.
   a. Potassium is more permeable than sodium
   b. Three sodium ejected for two potassium
   c. Potassium is brought into the cell and sodium expelled out of the cell
   d. All of the above
14. How much change of action potential can trigger a depolarization?
   a. 5 – 10 mv
   b. 10 – 15 mv
   c. 15 – 20 mv
   d. >25 mv
15. Usually various pulsed currents cause_____.
   a. Chemical changes
   b. Stimulate excitable tissue
   c. Heating in the tissue
   d. Changes in growth and repair in tissue
16. Before applying any electrical modality, the therapist should reason out_____.
   a. Whether the modality has the ability to achieve the intended effect?
   b. Is it safe?
   c. Is this the best modality for the particular effect
   d. All of the above

17. The essential for electromagnetic induction is _____.
    a. A conductor
    b. Magnetic lines of forces
    c. Movement of the conductor and magnetic lines of force relatively
    d. All of the above
18. To prevent the occurrence of eddy currents _____.
    a. An insulator is used
    b. A spherical conductor is used
    c. A laminated conductor is used
    d. None of the above
19. A choke coil is used _____.
    a. To even out the variations of intensity of current
    b. To prevent the flow of high frequency current and allow the flow of low frequency current
    c. (a) and (b)
    d. None of the above
20. The unit of capacitance is _____.
    a. Ampere   b. Volt
    c. Farad   d. None of the above
21. The low frequency current is up to
    a. 1000Hz   b. 50Hz
    c. 100Hz   d. None of the above
22. The duration of condenser discharge depends on _____.
    a. Capacitance and resistance
    b. Intensity of current
    c. Voltage
    d. None
23. Russian current is _____.
    a. Low frequency   b. Medium frequency
    c. High frequency   d. None of the above
24. All electromagnetic radiations have _____.
    a. Same velocity   b. Same wavelength
    c. Same frequency   d. None of the above
25. The name of the coil used to produce Faradic current in past was _____.
    a. Choke coil   b. Smart Bristow Faradic coil
    c. Induction coil   d. None of above

26. Pulse ration is the ratio of current or voltage required_____.
    a. By 110 ms and 30 ms pulse
    b. 1 ms and 30 ms pulse
    c. 1 ms and 10 ms pulse
    d. 1 ms and 100 ms pulse
27. Faradic current is ___.
    a. An alternating current
    b. A direct current
    c. Interrupted current
    d. Modified current
28. Galvanic current is ___.
    a. An alternating current
    b. A direct current
    c. Interrupted current
    d. Modified current
29. _____ current is used for the stimulation of innervated muscles.
    a. Faradic   b. Faradic type
    c. Surged faradic   d. Interrupted galvanic
30. Faradic current when applied_____.
    a. Recruit type I fibre followed by type II
    b. Recruit type II followed by type I
    c. Recruit type I alone
    d. Recruit type II alone
31. Electric pulse that stimulate a nerve should be _____.
    a. Rapid rising and duration less than 1ms
    b. Slow rising and duration less than 1ms
    c. Rapid rising and duration less than 100 ms
    d. None of the above
32. Which of the followings is an absolute contraindication for electrical stimulation?
    a. Pace maker.   b. Insensitive skin.
    c. Unconscious patient. d. Ischemic heart disease.
33. Which stimulator is more comfortable, safe but less accurate ?
    a. Constant current   b. Constant voltage
    c. Both   d. None of the above

34. The motor point of a muscle is found at_____.
    a. Proximal 2/3rd and distal one third of muscle belly
    b. Proximal 1/4th with distal 3/4th of muscle belly
    c. Proximal 1/3rd and distal 2/3rd of muscle belly
    d. 50% of muscle length
35. Nerve accommodation can be avoided by _____
    a. Surging the current
    b. Using varying current
    c. Using a varying current that rises and falls suddenly
    d. None of the above
36. The electrode which can easily depolarize the membrane of a nerve is __
    a. Positively charged
    b. Negatively charged
    c. Called indifferent electrode
    d. None of the above
37. The technique to stretch adhesion in a muscle is called _____.
    a. Faradism under pressure
    b. Faradic foot bath
    c. Faradism under tension
    d. None of the above
38. Due to acetylcholine hyperactivity_____.
    a. The rheobase of enervated tissue is less
    b. The rheobase of innervated tissue is less
    c. For innervated and denervated tissue it is same
    d. None of the above
39. The appropriate current to know tendon rupture _____.
    a. Faradic current   b. TENS
    c. Galvanic current   d. None of the above
40. 1 ms pulse of 1mA current would have _____.
    a. 1 coulomb   b. 1m coulomb
    c. 1m coulomb   d. None of the above
41. In a dynamic application of current which type of stimulation is preferable?
    a. Constant current   b. Constant voltage
    c. Both are preferred   d. None of them preferred

42. Long duration current can have a pulse duration_____.
    a. >1msec b. >1m sec
    c. 100 m sec d. 1 sec
43. Accommodation pulses can stimulate_____.
    a. Sensory nerve b. Motor nerve
    c. Muscles d. All of the above
44. Short duration currents have duration of_____.
    a. < 1 m sec b. < 1 m sec
    c. < 10 m sec d. < 10 m sec
45. Pulses of TENS are usually_____.
    a. Uniphasic
    b. Biphasic
    c. Biphasic with even charge
    d. Biphasic, even charge with equal or unequal pulse shape in both direction
46. Ab fibers stimulated by _____ TENS.
    a. High TENS b. Low TENS
    c. Both d. None of the above
47. Non-myelinated fiber is_____.
    a. Aa b. Ab
    c. Ag d. C
48. Depolarization of nerve occurs when the current is beyond threshold value about _____.
    a. 1 mv b. 10 mv
    c. 100 mv d. 1m v
49. In a rectangular pulse rheobase current a pulse duration of _____ can initiate a nerve impulse
    a. < 1 m sec b. < 0.5 m sec
    c. < 10 m sec d. < 100 m sec
50. Nociceptors are stimulated with a current intensity____.
    a. More than that stimulates sensory nerve
    b. More than that stimulate a motor nerve
    c. More than that cause tingling
    d. Less than that requires to produce a twitch
51. If the intensity remains constant at what frequency of current, the muscle contraction may decrease?
    a. < 100 Hz b. 100 Hz
    c. 1000 Hz d. < 1000 Hz

52. What is the optimal frequency for muscle contraction?
    a. 10 – 20 Hz b. 20 – 30 Hz
    c. 30 – 40 Hz d. 40 – 60 Hz
53. Fast twitch muscle fibers can be stimulated at a frequency of_____.
    a. 10 – 20 Hz b. 30 – 40 Hz
    c. 50 – 150 Hz d. 200 Hz
54. For a pulse duration of 1 ms what can be the maximum frequency for nerve depolarization_____.
    a. 100 Hz b. 500 Hz
    c. 1000Hz d. None of the above
55. Rhythmical 1 – 100 Hz interferential current may be helpful for_____.
    a. Muscle contraction b. Pain relief
    c. Reduction of edema d. None of the above
56. Benefit of Russian current over faradic stimulation is____.
    a. Better pain relieving effect
    b. Covers larger stimulation area
    c. Stimulation of deep muscles
    d. Better facilitator of healing
57. Which is a better electrotherapy modality for stress incontinence?
    a. TENS b. Faradic Stimulation
    c. IFT d. I.D.C
58. Skin impedance is _____.
    a. High for shorter pulse duration
    b. High for longer pulse duration
    c. Not affected by pulse duration
    d. High for high frequency current
59. Which one among the following is true for voluntary and electrical stimulation?
    a. Voluntary contraction stimulates type I but electrical stimulation stimulates type II fibres
    b. Voluntary stimulates type II but electrical stimulation type I
    c. There is gradual recruitment in electrical stimulation
    d. There is synchronized response in voluntary contraction

60. In the pre-mode application of IFT_____.
    a. Electrode placement is not easy
    b. Under the electrode current is more
    c. Difficult to accurately reach the affected area
    d. Strong contraction can not be achieved
61. What is the normal difference in current intensity between the two sides?
    a. < 2 mA   b. < 4 mA
    c. < 6 mA   d. < 8 mA
62. Beyond the conduction block in case of neurapraxia what should be the difference of current between two sides?
    a. < 2 mA   b. < 4 mA
    c. < 6 mA   d. < 8 mA
63. In unilateral nerve injury, when the required current intensity for stimulation is 10 – 20 times of opposite side normal muscle then what might be the condition?
    a. Neurapraxia
    b. Axonotemesis of few nerve fibers
    c. Axonotomesis of all most all nerve fibers
    d. Neurotemesis
64. What might be the strength of current required to stimulate a muscle with pulse of 10ms duration?
    a. Same as required for 30 ms pulse
    b. Same as required for 1 ms pulse
    c. Twice as 30 m sec pulse
    d. Half of 1 ms pulse
65. The rheobase is _____.
    a. Unchanged in a denervated muscle
    b. Increases in a denervated muscle
    c. Decreases in a denervated muscle
    d. First increase then decrease
66. Which among the following is correct for SD curve plotting?
    a. Constant current machine more comfortable
    b. Constant voltage machine is more comfortable
    c. Constant current comfortable and less accurate
    d. Constant voltage comfortable and less accurate

67. SD curve can_____.
   a. Distinguish between innervation and denervation
   b. Distinguish between innervated and denervated but can not quantify the state of innervation
   c. Distinguish innervated and denervated and quantify the state of innervation
   d. None
68. Chronaxie for denervated muscle is_____.
   a. < 1 ms   b. < 10 ms
   c. > 10 ms   d. > 1 ms
69. Rheobase is_____.
   a. Maximum tolerable current for a nerve impulse at long duration
   b. Minimum current for a nerve impulse at short duration
   c. Minimum current for a nerve impulse at long duration
   d. None of the above
70. Utilization time is_____.
   a. Same as chronaxie
   b. Pulse duration at rheobase current
   c. Shortest duration of pulse at rheobase current
   d. Longest duration of pulse at rheobase current
71. EMG reveals action potential of_____.
   a. Muscle   b. Motor unit
   c. Nerve fiber   d. None of the above
72. Which electrodes are used for more accurate EMG?
   a. Surface electrodes   b. Needle electrode
   c. Both   d. None
73. The physiological changes that occur during bio-feedback is due to _____.
   a. Unknown pathway
   b. known pathway
   c. Both
   d. None of the above
74. In EMG activities studied are_____.
   a. Insertional, spontaneous
   b. Insertional and exertional

c. Spontaneous and exertional
d. Insert ional, spontaneous and exertional

75. Which is a normal spontaneous activity?
    a. Fibrillation
    b. Positive sharp wave
    c. End phase spike
    d. None of the above
76. Which is not true for positive sharp wave?
    a. Diphasic potential
    b. Abrupt positive initial deflection
    c. Abrupt negative delay
    d. All of the above
77. What is not false about denervation potential?
    a. They appear 2-5 weeks after nerve injury
    b. They are present in primary muscle disease
    c. Includes fibrillation , fasciculation
    d. All of the above
78. Which is true for fasciculation?
    a. Spontaneous firing of the action potential of single muscle fibre
    b. None volitional random contraction of group of muscle fibre
    c. Duration 1-5 msec
    d. Frequency 1-50 Hz
79. The medium frequency current create a numbness, for which patient perceives a reduction in the intensity of current, is known as_____.
    a. Amplitude inhibition
    b. Current modulation
    c. Widensky inhibition
    d. None of the above
80. The chemical burn expected to occur due to passage of DC current into the body is likely to occur at_____.
    a. Cathode
    b. Anode
    c. Both the electrodes
    d. Where acids are formed
81. While applying DC, the important parameter for therapeutic purpose is_____.
    a. Current intensity
    b. Circuit resistance
    c. Current density
    d. The duration of application

82. In iontophoresis the total number of ions introduced into the tissue proportional to_____.
    a. Current
    b. Current density
    c. Time of application
    d. Both b and c
83. For iontophoresis the positively charged ions should be kept at_____.
    a. Anode
    b. Cathode
    c. Any electrode
    d. Both the electrodes
84. The factor/factors important for penetration of ion into the tissue is/are_____.
    a. Specific conductivity of solution
    b. pH of solution
    c. Precipitation formed by ions
    d. All of the above
85. The mechanism of wound healing by electrical stimulation is supposed to be due to_____.
    a. Skin battery
    b. Enhanced DNA and protein synthesis
    c. The migration of epithelial and connective tissue cells
    d. All of the above
86. What should be the sequence of application of current for an infected wound?
    a. Cathode on wound, < 1mA current, change of polarity of electrode
    b. Anode on wound, < 1mA current, change of polarity of electrode
    c. Cathode on wound, > 1mA current, change of polarity of electrodes
    d. Anode on wound, > 1mA current, change of polarity of electrode
87. The duration of anesthesia effect by application of anesthetic agent through iontophoresis is_____.
    a. 2 minutes
    b. < 5 minutes
    c. Within 15 minutes
    d. 20 minutes
88. What is the best therapeutic use of iontophoresis?
    a. As local anesthesia
    b. To apply antibiotics
    c. To apply anti inflammatory drug
    d. For treatment of hyperhydrosis

89. Which is not true for iontophoresis?
    a. Eliminates first pass metabolism
    b. Uncontrolled drug delivery
    c. Avoid pain that accompanies injection
    d. Decrease risk of infection.
90. Which iontophoresis is used for hyperhydrosis?
    a. Metallic silver
    b. Glycopyrronium bromide
    c. Xanthenes nicotinamide
    d. Vinc alkaloid
91. Zinc iontophoresis is used for _____.
    a. Neutrogena pain
    b. Ischemic ulcers
    c. Non healing ulcers
    d. Anti – inflammatory effect
92. Fungal skin infection can be treated by_____.
    a. Zinc iontophoresis
    b. Dexamethasone iontophoresis
    c. Copper iontophoresis
    d. Iodine iontophoresis
93. The principle of applying direct current to the body is_____.
    a. There should be uniform current density
    b. Provide a complete circuit
    c. The indifferent electrode size should be more than 2 ½ times the active electrode placed at therapeutic
    d. All of the above
94. The number of moles of a given ion that will be released by passage of current directly proportional to _____.
    a. Amperes of charge   b. Ejection time
    c. Transport number   d. a and b
    e. All of the above
95. Factors that affect the iontophoretic transport are _____.
    a. Concentration of various ions in the solution
    b. Vehicle pH
    c. Current strength
    d. Solute concentration
    e. All of the above

96. Among the following which is not true for application of iontophoresis_____.
    a. Low risk of infection
    b. Enhanced drug penetration
    c. Less systemic absorption
    d. Maximum skin irritation
97. For the edema reduction the following ion is used_____.
    a. Acetate   b. Copper
    c. Hyaluronidase   d. None of the above
98. What can be the source for iontophoresis in hyper hydrosis?
    a. Iodine   b. Acetic acid
    c. Zinc   d. Tap water
99. A typical iontophoretic drug delivery dose is_____.
    a. 20 mA – min   b. 40 mA – min
    c. 60 mA – min   d. 80 mA – min
100. If DC is used for pain relief the dosage varies with_____.
    a. Diagnosis of the condition
    b. Skin pigmentation
    c. Polarity of electrode on treatment site
    d. All of the above
101. Therapist should be cautious to treat patients with iontophoresis if they give history of _____.
    a. Skin reaction to histamine
    b. Dizziness
    c. Chronic headache
    d. All
102. For Calcific deposit , the ion selected is_____.
    a. Copper 50 – 60 C   b. Acetate
    c. Calciumd.   d. Magnesium
103. While treating hyperhydrosis in adults initially the dosage should be_____.
    a. >100 mA min   b. <100 mA min
    c. 200 mA min   d. 300 mA min
104. Chemical reaction increases by about _____ for each 1 C increase of tissue temperature
    a. 10 %   b. 20 %
    c. 14 %   d. 13 %

105. High frequency current when applied to the body produces_____.
    a. Motor stimulation
    b. Sensory stimulation
    c. Heat
    d. None of the above
106. Heat is produced in the body by the effect of _____.
    a. Low frequency current
    b. Medium frequency current
    c. High frequency current
    d. None of above
107. Which is not a deep heating modality?
    a. US   b. SWD
    c. MWD   d. HP
108. Cyclotherm apparatus is a _____.
    a. Heating modality   b. Cooling modality
    c. Both a and b   d. None
109. The temperature of PWB is _____.
    a. 30- 40 C   b. 40- 50 C
    c. 25- 55 C   d. None of the above
110. PWB is comfortable at 50^0 C temperatures, whereas water at 50^0 C temperature causes damage to skin, why?
    a. Low specific heat of PWB
    b. High specific heat of PWB
    c. High viscosity of PWB
    d. Latent heat of fusion of PWB
111. Region of thermal comfort is between_____.
    a. 45 – 5 C   b. 5 – 35 C
    c. 15 – 25 C   d. 5 – 45 C
112. The mode of heat transfer by hot pack, whirl pool bath, paraffin wax bath is___.
    a. conduction and convention
    b. conduction and radiation
    c. radiation and convention
    d. conduction, radiation and convention
113. The Hydrocollator packs are heated up to _____ temperature.
    a. 50 – 60 C   b. 75 – 80 C
    c. 40 – 50 C   d. None of the above

114. Which is superficial heating modality?
    a. Hydrocollator, wax bath, hydrotherapy and ultra sound.
    b. Electric heat pad, fluido therapy, short wave diathermy and infrared
    c. Hot pack, wax bath, hydrotherapy and infrared
    d. Microwave, hot pack, hydrotherapy and hot water bath
115. Heat is used prior to passive stretching exercises because of _____.
    a. Analgesic effect, reduction of viscosity and decrease collagen extensibility
    b. Analgesic effect, reduction of viscosity and increase collagen extensibility
    c. Analgesic effect, increase of viscosity and increase collagen extensibility
    d. Analgesic effect, increase of viscosity, sedative effect and reduction of muscle spasm
116. The loosing of heat from body by sweating is through _____.
    a. Conduction   b. Convection
    c. Radiation   d. None of the above
117. Heat is regulated by _____.
    a. Shivering
    b. Brown adipose tissue
    c. Sweating
    d. All of the above
118. Treatment by means of natural sunlight is called___.
    a. Actinotherapy
    b. Phototherapy
    c. Heliotherapy
    d. Radiating therapy
119. For which one among the following specific heat is highest
    a. Human body   b. Water
    c. Blood   d. Muscle
120. In wax bath the temperature is kept at a pre set temperature by using_____.
    a. Alcohol in glass thermometer

b. Thermostat
   c. Thermister
   d. None of the above
121. There is a circadian variation of body temperature of about_____.
    a. 1 degree C
    b. 2 degree C
    c. 1 degree F
    d. 2 degree F
122. Indiba treatment is modern version of _____.
    a. Short-wave diathermy
    b. Medium- wave diathermy
    c. Long- wave diathermy
    d. Inductothermy
123. When high frequency current is transmitted into the tissue, the molecules_____.
    a. Vibrate
    b. Oscillate
    c. Distort
    d. None of the above
124. The tissue that accumulates maximum heat with condenser field application of SWD is_____.
    a. Skin
    b. Fat
    c. Muscle
    d. Blood
125. The tissue heated most with cable method of SWD is _____.
    a. Periosteum
    b. Blood
    c. Bone
    d. Muscle
126. Dissipation of heat in SWD is maximized due to _____.
    a. Evaporation of sweat
    b. Air circulation
    c. Increased blood flow
    d. Contraction of muscle
127. In SWD most uniform field in the tissues is given by_____.
    a. Narrow spacing
    b. Wide spacing
    c. Medium spacing
    d. Even spacing
128. Therapeutic frequency of SWD is_____.
    a. 27.12 K Hz
    b. 27.12 MHz
    c. 27.12 G Hz
    d. None of the above
129. Sinuses are treated by SWD using ____ method.
    a. Coplanar
    b. Contraplanar
    c. Cross fire
    d. Monode

130. The beneficial effects of PSWD is in accordance with_____.
    a. Vant Hoffs rule	b. Joules law
    c. Arndt – Schultz law	d. None of the above
131. The frequency at which there is oscillation in the multivibrator circuit is_____.
    a. $f = 1/LC$	b. $1/2\Pi LC$
    c. $1/2\Pi L$	d. $1/2\Pi \sqrt{LC}$
132. During SWD application the treated part is included in the_____.
    a. Oscillator circuit	b. Resonator circuit
    c. Variable capacitor	d. None of the above
133. The depth of penetration of MWD lies_____.
    a. Between SWD and Infra red.
    b. Between SWD and PWB.
    c. Between SWD and US
    d. None of the above
134. Which of the following is the intermediate heating modality?
    a. IRR	b. MWD
    c. SWD	d. US
135. The approximate half value depth of penetration of Microwave is_____.
    a. 6 cm	b. 4 cm
    c. 3 cm	d. 1.5 cm
136. The depth of penetration of Microwaves is _____.
    a. Greater than Shortwaves
    b. Lesser than Infrared
    c. Greater than Infrared and lesser than Shortwaves
    d. None of the above
137. Microwaves are absorbed mostly in _____.
    a. Fat and fibrous tissues
    b. Bone
    c. Blood vessels
    d. Nerves
138. Superluminous diodes in LASER therapy is characterized by _____.
    a. Monochromatic, collimated, coherent
    b. Nonmonochromatic, collimated, coherent

c. Monochromatic, collimated, non-coherent
d. Monochromatic, non-collimated, coherent

139. LASER produces visible as well as infrared radiation, while infrared is strongly absorbed by _____.
    a. Water
    b. Haemoglobin
    c. Melanin
    d. Nervous tissue

140. What would be the energy density of laser therapy if mean power= 10mw, beam area = 1 cm and treatment time 30 sec
    a. 1 J/cm
    b. 3 J/cm.
    c. 0.3 J/cm.
    d. J/cm.

141. Which is not a neuropharmacological effect of laser for pain modulation?
    a. Alteration of serotonin metabolism
    b. Effect on collinergic system
    c. Opiate mediated
    d. Non-opiate mediated

142. For tennis elbow the laser dose is _____.
    a. 1.5 J/cm²
    b. 5 J/cm²
    c. 16-24 J/cm²
    d. 8-12 J/cm²

143. If pulse energy is 1 J, repetition rate is 10Hz, energy (laser) would be _____.
    a. 600J
    b. 60 J
    c. 10 J
    d. 1 J

144. Movement of drug through skin into subcutaneous tissue under the influence of Ultrasound is _____.
    a. Iontophoresis
    b. Phonophoresis
    c. Both
    d. None of the above

145. Ultrasound absorption is least in _____.
    a. Fat
    b. Blood
    c. Skin
    d. Bone

146. Which is not contraindication to US?
    a. Radiotherapy
    b. Haemoarthrosis
    c. First week after bony injury
    d. After laminectomy

147. Cavitation is _____.
    a. Thermal effects of US
    b. Non-thermal effects of US
    c. All the above
    d. None of the above
148. The characteristic of coupling medium are ———.
    a. High transmission properties, high viscosity, chemically inactive
    b. High transmission properties, high velocity, bubble formation
    c. Hypoallergic character, relative sterility and more difference in acoustic impedance between tissue and media
    d. Low viscosity, low transmission, high absorption properties.
149. The therapeutic range of ultrasound is_____.
    a. 1-5 Hz
    b. 5-10 Hz
    c. 0..5-5 MHz
    d. 0.5-100MHz
150. Pulsed treatment of ultrasound is given _____.
    a. For thermal effect
    b. For non-thermal effect
    c. Higher intensities can be given safely
    d. For chronic disease conditions
151. In ultrasound _____.
    a. The energy travels as waves.
    b. The energy pass as molecule
    c. The energy travels as matter
    d. None of the above
152. When the piezoelectric crystal change shape the parameter produced is_____.
    a. Amplitude of wave
    b. Frequency of the waves
    c. On and off pulses
    d. Wavelength of the wave
153. The velocity of ultrasound in a medium depends upon its_____.
    a. Density
    b. Elasticity

c. Both density and elasticity
d. Neither density nor elasticity.
154. What is the length of Fresnel zone in 3 cm diameter transducer working at 1MHz (wave length 1.5mm)?
   a. 10 cm
   b. 4.5 cm
   c. 15 cm
   d. 6 cm
155. In therapeutic ultrasound the energy travels _____.
   a. More in periphery of beam
   b. More in centre of the beam
   c. Uniform around the beam
   d. There is changing over from periphery to centre of beam.
156. Absorption of ultrasound is greatest in tissues with_____.
   a. Greatest water content and least structural protein content
   b. Greatest water and structural protein content
   c. Lowest water and structural protein content
   d. Greatest structural protein and lowest water content.
157. In the body the absorption of ultrasound is maximum in_____.
   a. Blood
   b. Nerve
   c. Skin
   d. Bone
158. Attenuation of ultrasound is due to _____.
   a. Reflection and refraction
   b. Absorption and scattering
   c. Reflection and absorption
   d. Scattering and refraction
159. For an ultrasound application output of $1W/cm^2$ how much will be the approximate temperature
   a. $1^0 c/min$
   b. $2^0 c/min$
   c. $3^0 c/min$
   d. $5^0 c/min$
160. For pulsed ultrasound application if the pulse length is 2ms and the interval is 8ms. What is the duty cycle?
   a. 25%
   b. 20%
   c. 10%
   d. None of the above
161. The purpose of application of pulsed ultrasound is to____.
   a. Dissipate the heat in the interval
   b. To produce higher mechanical effect

c. To lessen the thermal effect
  d. To lessen thermal effect and increase the mechanical effect.
162. What can produce transient cavitation?
  a. High intensity
  b. High frequency
  c. Continuous mode of ultrasound
  d. None of the above.
163. In the acute stage ultrasound has a _____.
  a. Anti-inflammatory effect
  b. Proinflammatory effect
  c. Vasodilatory and washing out effect
  d. Pain relieving effect
164. In the granulation stage U.S can _____.
  a. Promote collagen synthesis
  b. Enhance growth of capillaries
  c. Helps in proliferation of fibroblast
  d. All of the above
165. For stress fracture, therapeutic U.S is _____.
  a. Therapeutic
  b. Diagnostic
  c. Diagnostic and therapeutic
  d. Preventive
166. U.S may not be effective in _____.
  a. Soft tissue injury
  b. Bony injury
  c. Improving muscle blood flow
  d. Chronic pain.
167. Therapeutic ultrasound uses _____.
  a. Near field
  b. Far field
  c. Both near and far field
  d. More near field less far field
168. The ultrasound energy is more when _____.
  a. Frequency is high
  b. Amplitude is high
  c. Frequency and amplitude both are high
  d. Frequency low and amplitude is high

169. The relationship between penetration and absorption of ultrasound energy is
    a. Direct
    b. Inverse
    c. Linear
    d. None of the above
170. The approximate average half value depth of ultrasound of 1 M Hz frequency is _____.
    a. 100 mm
    b. 65 mm
    c. 35 mm
    d. 25 mm
171. The approximate average half value depth of ultrasound of 3 M Hz frequency is _____.
    a. 70mm
    b. 60 mm
    c. 30 mm
    d. 20 mm
172. Excessive dose of ultrasound causes periosteal pain which is mainly due to _____.
    a. Absorption
    b. Scattering
    c. Penetration
    d. Shear wave
173. During ultrasound application the head is moved to ____.
    a. Smooth out the irregularities of near field
    b. Reduce irregularities of absorption
    c. Both a and b
    d. None
174. By pulsing the ultrasound wave _____.
    a. Spatial average intensity is reduced
    b. Time average intensity is reduced
    c. Spatial peak temporal peak is reduced
    d. None of the above
175. To have effect on intracellular calcium system the ultrasound duty cycle should be _____.
    a. 10%
    b. 20%
    c. 30%
    d. 40%
176. The Maximum penetration depth of IR is _____.
    a. 3000 nm
    b. 1000 nm
    c. 700 nm
    d. 15000 nm
177. Depth of penetration of infrared of 3000nm wavelength is _____.
    a. 1 mm
    b. 3 mm
    c. 0.1 mm
    d. 2 mm

178. Infrared has a strong effect on_____.
    a. Bone
    b. Fat
    c. Skin
    d. None of the above
179. Infra red radiation has the wave length in between_____.
    a. Ultra violate and Visible radiation
    b. Micro wave diathermy and Visible radiation.
    c. Micro wave diathermy and Ultra violate radiation.
    d. Micro wave diathermy and Ultrasound
180. Penetration depth in Infra-red_____.
    a. 100% infrared absorbed
    b. 50% infrared absorbed
    c. 63% infrared absorbed
    d. 83% infrared absorbed
181. Infrared of 1000nm wave length can penetrate up to _____.
    a. Epidermis.
    b. Dermis.
    c. Muscle.
    d. Bone
182. In infrared radiation the frequency is_____.
    a. Directly proportional to the temperature
    b. Inversely proportional to the temperature
    c. Does not have any relation with temperature
    d. Directly proportional to the shape of the object
183. Human body emits _____.
    a. Infrared
    b. Microwave
    c. Ultrasound
    d. None of the above
184. Among the following electrotherapy modalities which is the right sequence of decreasing frequency?
    a. Infra red, ultrasound, short wave, interferential
    b. Infra red, microwave, short wave, interferential
    c. Ultraviolet, microwave, infrared, interferential
    d. Infrared, ultraviolet, microwave, medium frequency current
185. The local errythema after infrared radiation may lasts up to_____.
    a. 10 minutes
    b. 20 minutes
    c. 30 minutes
    d. 1 hour
186. At what distance should the infrared lamp of 750 watts be placed?
    a. 4 meter
    b. 6 meter
    c. 1 meter
    d. 1.5 meter

187. Which is not a contraindication of infrared?
    a. Psoriasis
    b. Defective arterial cutaneous circulation
    c. Dermatitis
    d. Defective blood pressure regulation
188. UVA is _____.
    a. Biotic
    b. Abiotic
    c. Germicidal
    d. None of the above
189. Epidermal transit time is about_____.
    a. 30 days
    b. 6 days
    c. 28 days
    d. 21 days
190. The UVR most effective in producing Vit.-D is_____.
    a. 400-313 nm
    b. 200-280 nm
    c. 280-300 nm
    d. None of the above
191. UV B & UV C are absorbed in _____.
    a. Cornea
    b. Lens of eye
    c. Both
    d. None of the above
192. Which law is applicable to determine the distance between ultraviolet source and skin?
    a. Inverse square law
    b. Bunsen-Roscoe raciprocity law
    c. Van't Hoff's law
    d. None of the above
193. Neonatal Jaundice can be treated by _____.
    a. Red light
    b. Blue light
    c. Infra red
    d. Yellow light
194. Prolonged application of UVR may produce skin cancers because_____.
    a. It damages melanocytes
    b. It damages keratinocytes
    c. It damages sebaceous glands
    d. It damages langerhans cells.
195. Which is not therapeutics effect of UVR?
    a. Reduction of blood pressure
    b. Treatment of acne valgaris
    c. Pain reduction
    d. Increased vitamin-D production

196. Treatment with UVR and visible radiation is _____.
    a. Helio therapy   b. Actino therapy
    c. Photo therapy   d. Photobiomodulation
197. Which UV radiation is/are abiotic _____.
    a. UVA   b. UVA and UVB
    c. UVC   d. UVA and UVC
198. Mostly UVR is absorbed in _____.
    a. Epidermis   b. Dermis
    c. Subcutaneous tissue   d. Capillary loop
199. E2 dose of UVR is _____.
    a. 2 X E1 dose   b. 2.5 X E1 dose
    c. 3 X E1 dose   d. 5 X E1 dose
200. Skin oedema occurs in ———— dose of UVR.
    a. E1   b. E2
    c. E3   d. E4
201. E3 dose of UVR can be given to ————% of body.
    a. 50%   b. 22%
    c. 11%   d. 4%
202. Erythema is best provoked by _____.
    a. UVA
    b. UVB
    c. UVC
    d. All provoke erythema to the same extent
203. Which one among the UVR can produce cataract?
    a. UVA
    b. UVB
    c. UVC
    d. All can produce cataract to the same extent
204. The strongest predictor for intramuscular cooling is _____.
    a. Skin temperature
    b. Adipose tissue thickness
    c. Room and core temperature
    d. Time
205. The systemic effects of cryotherapy is _____.
    a. Increased blood pressure
    b. Decreased blood pressure
    c. Decreased cardiac output
    d. None of the above

206. Cold induced vasodilatation is due to _____.
    a. Local neurogenic axon reflex
    b. Local release of vasodilator hormone
    c. Gradual paralysis of smooth muscles of vessels
    d. All of the above
207. Optimal temperature at which enzyme system for chemical and biological process operates is _____.
    a. 15 C   b. 21 C
    c. 27 C   d. 36 C
208. When the tissue temperature is 10 – 110C metabolism reduces by _____.
    a. 25%   b. 50%
    c. 75%   d. None of the above
209. Peripheral nerve fibres those are affected by cooling in order are _____.
    a. A ä,Aâ, Aã
    b. Aâ, Aã, C
    c. B, C , Aã
    d. All the fibres are equally affected
210. Joint position sense is affected by cryotherapy upto_____.
    a. 5 minutes   b. 10 minutes
    c. Up to 15 minutes d. 30 minutes
211. To have neuromuscular effect of cryotherapy the application should be upto _____.
    a. 20 minutes   b. 30 minutes
    c. 45 minutes
    d. None of the above
212. For facilitation brisk icing duration is _____.
    a. 1 second   b. 2 second
    c. 3 second   d. 4 second
213. Spasticity can be reduced by_____.
    a. Heating   b. Cooling
    c. SWD   d. TENS
214. Kaolin has been used as_____.
    a. Hot moist pack b. Dry hot pack
    c. Cold pack   d. UV
215. Evaporating spray used in sports injury, contains_____.
    a. Fluori methane. b. Fluori ethane.
    c. Chlori ethane.   d. Ethyl chloride.

216. Fluido therapy contains_____.
    a. Warm water in large cabinet.
    b. Water in room temp in large cabinet.
    c. Cold water in large cabinet.
    d. Mass of tiny cellulose particles suspended in moving air
217. Under cold condition the blood flow to each 100 gms of skin can be reduced to minimum about_____.
    a. 2 ml/ min
    b. 20 ml/ min
    c. 30 ml/ min
    d. 1 ml/ min.
218. Which fibers are least affected by ice?
    a. C fiber
    b. Delta fiber
    c. Aâ fiber
    d. A Gamma fiber
219. Which therapeutic effect will differentiate between cold and heat treatments?
    a. Relieving pain
    b. Reduction of spasticity
    c. Reduction of spasm
    d. None of above
220. The extent of reduction in tissue temperature following cryotherapy depend on_____.
    a. Nature of substance applied and region of the body to which it is applied
    b. Temperature difference between the substance and the skin
    c. Duration of application
    d. All of the above

ANSWER SHEET ELECTROTHERAPY

1. a	2. d	3. d	4. d	5. d
6. b	7. d	8. a	9. d	10. d
11. b	12. d	13. d	14. b	15. d
16. d	17. d	18. c	19. c	20. c
21. a	22. a	23. b	24. a	25. b
26. d	27. a	28. b	29. c	30. a

31. a	32. a	33. b	34. c	35. c
36. b	37. c	38. a	39. a	40. b
41. b	42. b	43. c	44. a	45. d
46. a	47. d	48. b	49. a	50. b
51. b	52. c	53. c	54. b	55. c
56. c	57. c	58. b	59. a	60. b
61. a	62. a	63. c	64. c	65. c
66. b	67. c	68. c	69. c	70. c
71. b	72. b	73. a	74. d	75. c
76. c	77. c	78. c	79. c	80. a
81. c	82. d	83. a	84. a	85. d
86. d	87. c	88. d	89. b	90. b
91. b	92. c	93. d	94. e	95. e
96. d	97. c	98. d	99. b	100. d
101. d	102. b	103. b	104. d	105. c
106. c	107. d	108. c	109. b	110. a
111. c	112. a	113. b	114. c	115. b
116. b	117. d	118. c	119. b	120. b
121. a	122. c	123. c	124. b	125. b
126. c	127. c	128. b	129. c	130. c
131. d	132. b	133. a	134. b	135. c
136. c	137. c	138. c	139. a	140. c
141. c	142. c	143. a	144. b	145. b
146. c	147. b	148. a	149. c	150. b
151. a	152. b	153. c	154. c	155. b
156. d	157. d	158. b	159. a	160. b
161. b	162. a	163. b	164. d	165. b
166. c	167. a	168. c	169. b	170. b
171. c	172. d	173. c	174. b	175. b
176. b	177. c	178. c	179. b	180. c
181. b	182. a	183. a	184. b	185. c
186. b	187. a	188. a	189. c	190. c
191. a	192. a	193. b	194. d	195. d
196. c	197. c	198. a	199. a	200. c
201. d	202. c	203. a	204. d	205. a
206. d	207. c	208. b	209. a	210. c
211. b	212. d	213. b	214. a	215. a
216. d	217. d	218. a	219. b	220. d

CHAPTER 3

Physiotherapy in Orthopaedic Conditions

1. The term orthopaedic is derived from Greek words, which means____
   a. Art of preventing and correcting deformities in children
   b. Art of managing fracture and dislocation
   c. Dealing with diseases and injuries of the trunk and limbs
   d. Dealing with diseases and injuries of bones, joints, muscles and ligaments
2. Green stick fracture is seen in_____.
   a. Adult   b. Children
   c. At any age   d. Elderly
3. With fractures of the shaft of long bones, rotation is controlled by ___.
   a. Immobilizing the joint close to the fracture site in slight flexion
   b. Immobilizing the joint close to the fracture site in neutral position
   c. Immobilizing the joints above and below it
   d. Surgery

4. External fixation is used for ____.
   a. Fracture with severe soft tissue injury involving skin and blood vessels
   b. Unstable fracture
   c. Pathological fracture
   d. Multiple fractures
5. Burst fracture is seen in_____.
   a. Talus fracture
   b. Vertebral fracture
   c. Femoral head fracture
   d. Scaphoid
6. Plaster of paris is_____.
   a. Hemihydrated calcium sulphate
   b. Hemihydrated calcium carbonate
   c. Hemihydrated calcium bicarbonate
   d. None of the above
7. The epiphyseal plate is a barrier to the spread of infection, but if the involved metaphyses lie wholly or partly within a joint cavity, the joint is liable to become infected. Which of the following metaphysic is not intra-capsular?
   a. Upper metaphysis of humerus
   b. Upper and lower metaphyses of femur
   c. All the metaphyses at the elbow
   d. Lower metaphysic of tibia
8. Ricket is due to deficiency of_____.
   a. Vit A   b. Vit B
   c. Vit C   d. Vit D
9. Brodies abscess is a form of_____.
   a. Acute osteomyelitis
   b. Chronic osteomyelitis.
   c. Tubercular osteomyelitis
   d. Syphilis
10. Glenoid faces _____
    a. Laterally downward,
    b. Forward, upward and laterally
    c. Backward, downward, outward
    d. Forward, downward and medially

11. Head of the humerus measures almost half a sphere with an angular value _____
    a. 180 degrees   b. 160 degrees
    c. 150 degrees   d. 120 degrees
12. Neck shaft angle of humerus is _____
    a. 45 degrees   b. 60 degrees
    c. 90 degrees   d. 120 degrees
13. At rest scapula makes an angle of about _____ with the frontal plane.
    a. 15 degrees   b. 30 degrees
    c. 45 degrees   d. 60 degrees
14. Scapulo clavicular angle at rest is about _____
    a. 30 degrees   b. 45 degrees
    c. 60 degrees   d. 90 degrees
15. Root of spine of scapula corresponds to _____
    a. T2.   b. T3
    c. T5   d. T7
16. Glenohumeral joint capsule is laxed to allow mobility. The head of the humerus can be detracted laterally about _____ with the arm by the side
    a. 2 cm   b. 3 cm
    c. 4 cm   d. 5 cm
17. _____ checks the downward pull of gravity on the arm by the side
    a. Superior joint capsule
    b. Rotator cuff
    c. Glenohumeral ligament
    d. Deltoid
18. External rotation of glenohumeral joint is checked by _____
    a. Middle glenohumeral ligament
    b. Inferior glenohumeral ligament
    c. Anterior coracohumeral ligament
    d. Posterior coracohumeral ligament
19. Trapezoid ligament of acromio clavicular joint checks _____
    a. Medical movement of clavicle
    b. Lateral movement of clavicle

c. Downward movement
d. Upward movement.
20. _____ rotates the clavicle backward during elevation
   a. Upper trapezius   b. Trapezoid ligament
   c. Conoid ligament   d. Deltoid.
21. Elevation of medial end of clavicle at sternoclavicular joint is checked by _____
   a. Anterior costoclavicular ligament
   b. Posterior costoclavicualr ligament
   c. Superior costoclavicular ligament
   d. Inferior costoclavicular ligament
22. _____ bursa often communicates with the shoulder joint
   a. Subacromial bursa   b. Subscapular bursa
   c. Subdeltoid bursa   d. None
23. In kyphotic posture _____ is responsible for the stability of glenohumeral joint with the arm by the side
   a. Tension of superior gleno humeral capsule
   b. Coracohumeral ligament
   c. Rotator cuff
   d. Deltoid
24. _____ is the closed pack position of shoulder joint.
   a. Abduction and external rotation
   b. Flexion and external rotation
   c. Horizontal abduction and external rotation
   d. None
25. Resting position of gleno humeral joint is _____
   a. 30 degrees of abduction and 30 degrees of flexion and some external rotation
   b. 60 degrees of abduction and 30 degrees of horizontal abduction
   c. 45 degrees of abduction and 30 degrees of flexion and some internal rotation
   d. 30 degrees of abduction and 60 degrees of horizontal abduction
26. Capsular pattern of shoulder joint is _____.
   a. Restriction of lateral rotation
   b. Restriction of rotation and flexion

c. Restriction of external rotation and abduction
   d. Decrease of external rotation
27. The commonest structures impinged is _____
   a. Infraspinatus   b. Supraspinatus
   c. Long head of biceps   d. Subacromial bursa
28. Physiotherapy for shoulder impingement syndrome includes____.
   a. Restoration of shoulder external rotation and scapular rotation
   b. Balancing deltoid-ratator cuff and trapezius-serratus anterior force couples
   c. Managing ACJ degenerative arthritis
   d. All of the above
29. Locking position of shoulder joint is
   a. Flexion, abduction and internal rotation
   b. External rotation, abduction and internal rotation
   c. Extension, abduction, external rotation
   d. Flexion, abduction, external rotation.
30. Drop arm test indicates _____
   a. Weakness of deltoid   b. Rupture of suprasinatus
   c. Positive painful arc   d. None
31. A patient of frozen shoulder has 30 degrees of external rotation. Which mobilization technique would be indicated with such a limitation?
   a. Lateral distraction and anterior glide
   b. Lateral distraction and posterior glide
   c. Medial distraction and posterior glide
   d. Medial distraction and inferior glide
32. When evaluating a case of bicipital tendonitis which clinical finding you would NOT expect to find _____
   a. Increase in pain on isometric resistance to biceps
   b. Referred pain in C7, C8 dermatomes
   c. Painful arc with AROM
   d. Tenderness over bicipital tendon.
33. A patient is referred to you after three weeks of immobilization of shoulder following a dislocation. You may begin treatment with all of the following except _____
   a. Isometric shoulder exercises
   b. Passive ROM exercises

c. Active resisted ROM exercises
d. Isokinetic exercise with high speed.
34. Post operative physiotherapy following fracture clavicle includes___.
    a. Active free shoulder movements
    b. Avoidance of elevation and lifting weight
    c. Shoulder rotation mobilization
    d. All of the above
35. Fracture shaft humerus is associated with
    a. Axillary nerve injury
    b. Radial nerve injury
    c. Brachial plexus injury.
    d. Median nerve injury
36. Post operative physiotherapy following Putti-platt surgery for anterior recurrent shoulder dislocation are
    a. Isometric contraction of rotator cuff after surgery
    b. Active movements can be started after 3-4 week
    c. Mobilization of shoulder can be started after 3-4 weeks
    d. Progressive strengthening can be started after 3-4 weeks
37. ACJ injury can be managed by strengthening ___ muscles.
    a. Rotator cuff and deltoid
    b. Deltoid and trapezius
    c. Trapezius and serratus anterior
    d. Rotator cuff and serratus anterior
38. Positive adson's test indicates TOS due to___.
    a. Scalene   b. Cervical rib
    c. Reduced scapuloclavicular angle
    d. Tumour
39. Physiotherapy for thoracic outlet syndrome includes___.
    a. Stretching of Scalenei, levator scapulae and pectorals to relieve pressure
    b. Strengthening of trapezius and serratus anterior to correct posture
    c. Modalities like US, moist heat to relive spasm and TENS, IFT to relieve pain
    d. All of the above

40. Close packed position for humeroulnar joint is
    a. extension
    b. 50 degrees of flexion
    c. 70 degrees of flexion
    d. 90 degrees of flexion
41. Resting position for humeral radial joint is _____
    a. Semiflexion and supinaton
    b. Semiflexion and pronation
    c. Extension and supination
    d. Extension and pronation
42. Capsular pattern of limitation of elbow joint is _____
    a. Limitation of flexion
    b. Limitation of flexion more than extension
    c. Limitation of extension more than flexion
    d. Limitation of extension
43. Extension of elbow is associated with _____
    a. Ulnar abduction and forearm pronation
    b. Ulnar abduction and supination of forearm
    c. Inferior glide of ulna
    d. Superior glide of radius
44. Flexion of elbow is associated with
    a. Inferior glide of ulnar and superior glide of radius
    b. Superior glide of ulna and inferior glide of radius
    c. Ulnar abduction and forearm pronation
    d. Radial adduction and forearm pronation
45. Usually the direction of elbow dislocation is _____.
    a. Backward
    b. Backward and lateral
    c. Backward and medial
    d. Forward
46. Following fracture supracondylar of humerus the small distal fracture segment is displaced backward. Uncorrected displaced fracture will limit _____ movement.
    a. Elbow flexion   b. Elbow extension
    c. Forearm rotation
    d. Alter carrying angle

47. Tennis elbow may involve___
    a. Common extensors origin characterized by pain during resisted isometric contraction
    b. Radio-humeral or superior radio-ulnar joint characterized by pain during joint play
    c. Lateral collateral ligament or annular ligament characterized by pain during passive movements, joint play and stress test
    d. All of the above
48. Typical tennis elbow involves the common extensor muscles. Which muscle is commonly involved?
    a. Extensor carpi radialis longus
    b. Extensor carpi radialis bravis
    c. Brachioradialis
    d. Extensor Indices
49. VIC following fracture supracondylar of humerus results from____.
    a. Injury to brachial artery by the projected sharp proximal segment of humerus
    b. Tight plaster
    c. Excessive elbow flexion during immobilization
    d. All of the above
50. Distal articulating surface of radius faces _____
    a. Inferiorly   b. Palmarly and ulnarly
    c. Dorsally and ulnarly   d. Palmarly and outward
51. The carpal tunnel dimension increases with _____
    a. Wrist flexion   b. In neutral
    c. In extension   d. None
52. There are _____ long bones in hand
    a. 15   b. 17
    c. 19   d. 22
53. There are _____ joints that make up the hand complex
    a. 17   b. 19
    c. 21   d. 27
54. The carpo metacarpal joint of little finger is having _____ degrees of freedom
    a. 1   b. 2
    c. 3   d. none

55. Mallet finger is due to _____
    a. Contracture of FDP
    b. Rupture of collateral slip of extensor expansion
    c. Rupture of central slip of extensor expansion
    d. Rupture of the volar plate
56. Swan neck deformity is due to _____
    a. Contracture of extensor digitorum communis
    b. Intrinsic tightness
    c. Contracture of FDP
    d. Rupture/laxity of volar plate.
57. Bouttenaire deformity is due to _____
    a. Contracture of FDS
    b. Rupture of central slip of extensor expansion
    c. Contracture of extensor digitorum
    d. Rupture of collateral slip of extensor expansion
58. Intrinsic tightness is characterized by _____
    a. Increased DIP joint extension with PIP flexion than that with PIP joint extension
    b. Increased IP joint flexion with MCP joint flexion than that with MCP joint extension
    c. Increased IP joint flexion with wrist flexion than that with wrist extension
    d. None
59. Tightness oblique retinacular ligament is characterized by _____
    a. Decreased DIP joint flexion with PIP flexion than that with PIP extension
    b. Decreased DIP flexion with PIP extension than that with PIP flexion
    c. Decreased IP joint flexion with MCP joint flexion than that with MCP joint extension
    d. Decreased IP joint flexion with wrist flexion than that with wrist extension
60. The MCP joint is stable in _____
    a. Semi flexion   b. Maximum flexion
    c. Extension   d. Hyperextension
61. The capsule, collateral ligaments, and accessory collateral ligaments of the MCP joints are taut in its close

packed position, which is the closed packed position of MCP joint?
a. 40 degree of flexion   b. Maximum flexion
c. Neutral   d. Hyperextension

62. Hyperextension at IP joint of finger is checked by
    a. Volar plate   b. PDS
    c. Tension of the skin   d. Collateral ligament

63. Inflammation of sheath of the_____ tendons within the sheath is referred as Dequervein's disease.
    a. FPL and FPB
    b. ERL and EPB
    c. Abductor pollicis longus and abductor pollicis brevis
    d. Abductor pollicis longus and extensor pollicis brevis

64. The space between _____ and _____ is referred to as Noman's land.
    a. PIP joint and DIP joint
    b. MCP joint and PIP joint
    c. MCP joint and DIP joint
    d. Wrist joint to MCP joint

65. Close packed position for the wrist is _____
    a. Neutral
    b. Full Dorsiflexion with radial deviation
    c. Full flexion
    d. 45 degrees of dorsiflexion with ulnar deviation

66. The transverse metacarpal arch increases with
    a. Clenched fist
    b. Opening the fist
    c. Thumb opposition
    d. None

67. During wrist extension _____
    a. Distal carpals glides palmarly
    b. Proximal carpals glides palmarly
    c. Proximal carpal glide dorsally
    d. Proximal carpals supinates on radius

68. The capsular pattern of wrist joint is _____
    a. More limitation of wrist extension than flexion
    b. Equal limitation of wrist extension and flexion
    c. More limitation of wrist flexion than extension
    d. More limitation of ulnar deviation than radial deviation

69. The resting position for wrist is _____
    a. 30 degrees of extension with radial deviation
    b. 30 degrees of extension with neutral deviation
    c. Neutral extension with slight ulnar deviation
    d. 10 degrees of flexion
70. Component motion of MCP joint flexion include _____
    a. Dorsal gliding, pronation, ulnar deviation and distraction of base of proximal phalanx.
    b. Palmar gliding, supination, ulnar deviation and approximation of base of proximal phalanx on metacarpal
    c. Dorsal gliding, supination, ulnar deviation and approximation of base of proximal phalanx.
    d. Palmar gliding, pronation, radial deviation and distraction of base of proximal phalanx.
71. Component motion of IP flexion of fingers include _____
    a. Dorsal glide, pronation, ulnar deviation & distraction of more distal phalanx on the head of the proximal phalanx.
    b. Palmar glide, pronation, ulnar deviation, approximation of distal phalanx on the head of the proximal phalanx.
    c. Dorsal glide, supination, radial deviation, approximation, distal phalanx on the head of the proximal phalanx.
    d. Palmar glide, supination, radial deviation and distraction of more distal phalanx, on head of proximal phalanx.
72. Avascular necrosis of scaphoid fracture occurs at
    a. Proximal half   b. Distal half
    c. Whole bones   d. None of the above
73. Reverse colle's fracture is otherwise known as
    a. Barton's fracture   b. Smith fracture
    c. Galeazzi fracture   d. Pott's fracture
74. Following extensor tendon repair in the hand ____.
    a. The involved finger is only immobilized

b. All the fingers are immobilized
c. Adjacent fingers are immobilized
d. None of the above
75. Angle of inclination of femur refers to
    a. Neck shaft angle in saggital plane.
    b. Neck shaft angle in frontal plane
    c. Neck shaft angle in transverse plane
    d. None
76. Neck shaft angle in femur in frontal plane in child is _____

    a. 120 degreees   b. 130 degrees
    c. 150 degrees   d. 170 degrees
77. Neck shaft angle of femur in transverse plane is referred as _____
    a. Angle of inclination   b. Angle of anteversion
    c. Angle of declination   d. Coxa valga
78. Increase in angle of inclination of femur is referred to as
    a. Coxa valga   b. Coxa plane
    c. Coxa vara   d. Anteversion
79. Increase in torsion angle of femur is referred to as _____

    a. Coxa valga   b. Coxa vara
    c. Anteversion   d. Retroversion
80. In toeing gait is the characteristic feature of _____
    a. Coxa valga   b. Coxa vara
    c. Anteversion   d. Retroversion
81. Reduced internal rotation of hip is the feature of _____

    a. Coxa valga   b. Coxa vara
    c. Anteversion   d. Retroversion
82. The bending moment in the neck of femur is increased predisposing to the fracture neck in _____
    a. Coxa valga   b. Coxa vara
    c. Anteversion   d. Retroversion
83. The tip of greater trochanter lies above the shenton's line in _____
    a. Coxa valga   b. CDH
    c. Anteversion   d. None of the above

84. The stable position for the hip is _____
    a. Flexion, external rotation and abduction
    b. Extension, external rotation and adduction
    c. Neutral extension, internal rotation and abduction
    d. Full flexion, internal rotation and adduction
85. _____ strongest ligament in the body
    a. Ischiofemoral   b. Round ligament
    c. Pubofemoral   d. Iliofemoral
86. One can hang on ilio femoral ligament using minimum muscle action by _____
    a. Rolling the pelvis backward
    b. Rolling the pelvis forward
    c. Extension, abduction and internal rotation of hip
    d. Extension, abduction, external rotation of hip
87. In neutral standing position the hip joint is weaker _____
    a. Anteriorly   b. Posteriorly
    c. Inferiorly   d. Superiorly
88. The resting position for the hip is _____
    a. Neutral extension, abduction and rotation
    b. 30 degrees of flexion, 30 degrees of abduction and slight external rotation
    c. Neutral extension, 30 degrees of abduction and slight internalrotation
    d. 30 degrees of flexion, slight adduction and internal rotation.
89. Capsular pattern of restriction of hip is _____
    a. Internal rotation and abduction most restricted, flexion and extension restricted
    b. External rotation and abduction most restricted, flexion and extension restricted
    c. Extension, internal rotation most restricted, flexion and external rotation restricted
    d. Flexion, internal rotation most restricted, extension and external rotation restricted.
90. The component motion for hip flexion is _____
    a. Inferior and lateral glide of femoral head in acetabulum
    b. Posterior and superior glide of femoral head in acetabulum

c. Posterior and inferior glide of femoral head in acetabulum
   d. Anterior and superior glide of femoral head in acetabulum
91. In single leg standing hip joint is subjected to load equal to _____
   a. 1/3rd of body weight
   b. body weight
   c. 2 times of body weight
   d. 3 times of body weight
92. In case of LLD _____ side bears more load
   a. Shorter
   b. Longer
   c. Both sides bears equal load
   d. None
93. In case of coxa vara _____ side is prone to develop degenerative arthritis
   a. Affected
   b. Unaffected
   c. Both
   d. None of the above.
94. Hip joint is supplied by _____ segments
   a. L1 – L3   b. L2 – L5
   c. L2 – S1   d. L3 – S2.
95. _____ bursa often communicates with the hip joint
   a. Subtrochantric   b. Ischeal
   c. Iliopectineal   d. Adductor
96. In case of hip arthritis patient often complain pain on _____ aspect of hip joint
   a. Anterior   b. Posterior
   c. Lateral   d. Medial
97. Lateral hip pain is the characteristic feature of _____
   a. Sciatica
   c. IT friction syndrome
   d. Hip arthritis

98. Pain in the buttock is suggestive of pain of _____ origin
    a. Lumbar spine   b. Hip spine
    c. Piriformis   d. Trochanteric
99. The characteristic features of slipped capital femoral epiphysis are _____.
    a. Limitation of abduction and internal rotation, femur rolls into abduction and external rotation during flexion and shortening.
    b. Limitation of flexion, abduction and internal rotation and shortening.
    c. Limitation of flexion and internal rotation, femur rolls into abduction and external rotation during flexion and lengthening
    d. Limitation of flexion, abduction and internal rotation and slengthening
100. Slipped capital femoral epiphysis occurs at _____ age
    a. Birth   b. 5 – 10 years
    c. 11 – 15 years   d. 16 – 20 years
101. Factors influencing prognosis in Perthe's disease includes ____.
    a. Early onset poor is the prognosis
    b. Early loss of hip movements poor is the pognosis
    c. Early weight bearing better is the prognosis
    d. Lateral sublaxation/ extrusion better is the prognosis
102. The principles of management of perthe's disease is___.
    a. Improve circulation to the femoral capital epiphysis
    b. Traction
    c. Containment, weight relieve and ROM
    d. Surgery
103. _____ splint is recommended for CDH.
    a. Pavlic harness   b. HKAFO
    c. DB Splint   d. Aeroplane
104. Backward lurching of trunk during stance phase suggest _____
    a. Hip extensor weakness on the side of swing leg
    b. Hip flexor weakness on the side of stance legs

c. Hip extensor weakness on the side of stance leg
   d. Hip abductor weakness on the side of stance legs
105. Antalgic gait is characterized by _____
   a. Smaller step on the affected side
   b. Smaller step on the sound side
   c. Lurching on the sound side
   d. Inadequate swing on the affected side
106. Pelvic inclination with the affected side upward implies _____
   a. Flexor contracture
   b. Abductor contracture
   c. Adductor contracture
   d. Adductor weakness
107. In Thomas test position limitation of hip adduction ROM is due to shortening of_____
   a. Iliopsoas
   b. TFL
   c. Rectus femoris
   d. Piriformis
108. Ely's test is done to check length of _____ muscle
   a. ITB
   b. Hamstrings
   c. Rectus femoris
   d. Hip adductors
109. Baer's SI point refers to a point located approximately on the spino umbilical line
   a. 2" from ASIS
   b. 2" from umbilical
   c. At the junction of medial 1/3rd and distal 2/3rd
   d. None of the above
110. The source of pain in OA of hip is _____
   a. Articular cartilage
   b. Joint capsule
   c. Muscles
   d. All of the above
111. _____ may give rise to secondary OA of hip
   a. LLD
   b. Capsular tightness

c. Fixed flexion deformity
d. All of the above

112. 1 KG increase in body weight adds _____ to the supporting femoral head during stance phase
    a. ½ Kg b. 1 kg
    c. 2 kg d. 3kg

113. In early OA pain is felt _____.
    a. Following activities due to fatigue
    b. Continuously due to inflammation
    c. Constant pain
    d. Night pain

114. The primary therapeutic goal in OA is _____.
    a. Relief by application of modalities
    b. Prevent further progression by stretching of the joint capsule
    c. Avoid weight bearing activities.
    d. Strengthening the muscles surrounding the joint

115. In fracture neck of femur the blood supply to the head of the femur is retained by _____.
    a. Circumflex artery
    b. Nutritient artery.
    c. Artery to ligament of the head of femur
    d. Femoral artery

116. Which of the following is the cause of avascular necrosis of head of femur following fracture neck _____.
    a. Severing of arteries supplying the head of femur
    b. Intracapsular joint effusion prevents haematoma formation following fracture
    c. Lack of soft tissue contact at the fracture site
    d. All of the above.

117. Complications of central fracture dislocation of hip joint _____.
    a. Intrapelvic haemmorrhage due to damage to vessels
    b. Genito-urinary tract damage
    c. Recurrent dislocation
    d. a and b

118. Characteristic features of traumatic posterior dislocation of hip_____.
    a. Fixed in adduction and internal rotation, limited JROM and shortening

b. Fixed in abduction and external rotation, limited JROM and shortening
c. Limited abduction and internal rotation and no limb length discrepancy
d. Fixed in adduction and external rotation, limited JROM and no limb length discrepancy

119. The primary indication of joint replacement is _____.
    a. Effusion
    b. Limited range of motion
    c. Muscle atrophy
    d. Pain

120. In case of THR, all of the following are true except____.
    a. Avoid flexion beyond 90, adduction beyond neutral and rotation
    b. Rolling through sound side
    c. Standing through affected side
    d. Leg swing in half standing

121. Which advice would not be correct for a patient following THR?
    a. When turning pivot to the affected side
    b. Do not cross your legs and keep a pillow between your legs while sleeping.
    c. Avoid low chairs
    d. All of the above

122. Replacement arthroplasty is a salvage procedure, the complications of which are instability and shortening. The post-operatively immobilization is given by skeletal traction for about 6 weeks and the physiotherapy includes___.
    a. Hip movements as pain allows
    b. Non weight bearing crutch walking and weight bearing allowed as good fibrous union occurs
    c. Strengthening exercises, weight relieving orthosis, foot wear compensation and walking aids
    d. All of the above

123. In standing tibio femoral angle in the frontal plane is about _____.
    a. 0 degrees
    b. 10 degrees
    c. 140 degrees
    d. 170 degrees

124. The articulating surface of patella consists of _____ facets.
    a. One   b. Two
    c. Three   d. Four
125. Medial meniscus forms _____.
    a. half of a large circle   b. almost all of a circle
    c. ᵗʰ of a circle   d. none
126. The function of meniscus is _____.
    a. shock absorber   b. lubrication nutrition
    c. load distribution   d. all
127. Medial meniscus is more prone to injury than lateral because_____.
    a. It is relatively more mobile.
    b. It is less mobile than lateral meniscus
    c. Medial compartment bears more than the lateral
    d. None of the above
128. MCL is _____.
    a. Long, Flat band   b. Short and rounded
    c. Short and flat bone   d. Long and rounded
129. MCL checks _____.
    a. Knee extension, abduction of tibia and external rotation
    b. Knee extension, abduction of tibia and internal rotation
    c. Knee flexion, adduction of tibia and internal rotation
    d. Knee flexion, abduction of tibia and external rotation
130. Lateral Collateral Ligament checks _____.
    a. Knee extension adduction of tibia and internal rotation
    b. Knee extension, adduction of tibia and external rotation
    c. Flexion abduction and external rotation
    d. Flexion adduction and internal rotation
131. ACL runs from the intercondylar area of the tibia _____.
    a. Forward, upward and medially
    b. Forward, upward and laterally
    c. Backward, upward and laterally
    d. Backward, upward and medially

132. ACL checks _____.
   a. Flexion, forward movement of tibia and external rotation
   b. Flexion, backward movement of tibia and internal rotation
   c. Extension, forward movement of tibia and internal rotation
   d. Extension, backward movement of tibia and external rotation
133. PCL checks _____.
   a. Backward movement of tibia, internal rotation and extension
   b. Backward movement of tibia, external rotation and flexion
   c. Forward movement of tibia, external rotation and extension
   d. Forward movement of tibia, internal rotation and flexion
134. Pes anserinus includes _____.
   a. Semimembranosus, gracilis and sartorius
   b. Semi membranosus, rectus femoris and ITB
   c. Semitendinosus, gracilis and sartorius
   d. Semitendinouss, pectineus and adductor magnus
135. Biceps femoris reinforces _____.
   a. Anterior cruciate ligament and LCL
   b. Posterior cruciate ligament and LCL
   c. Posterior cruciate ligament and MCL
   d. Anterior cruciate ligament and MCL
136. In case of MCL injury strengthening of _____ should be given.
   a. Pes anserinus and semi membranosus
   b. Hamstrings
   c. Hip adductors
   d. Quadriceps
137. House maid's knee refers to _____
   a. Infrapatellar bursitis   b. Prepatellar bursitis
   c. Suprapatellar bursitis   d. Quadriceps tendonitis

138. Knee extension is limited by _____
    a. Bony contact
    b. Tension of hamstrings
    c. Tension of posterior skin
    d. The tension of joint capsule
139. The closed packed position for the knee is _____
    a. Extension
    b. Full flexion
    c. 25 degrees of knee flexion
    d. 90 degrees of knee flexion
140. The capsular pattern of the knee is _____
    a. Flexion is more restricted than extension
    b. Extension is more restricted than flexion
    c. Flexion terminally restricted and extension full
    d. Extension terminally restricted and flexion full
141. The component motions of knee flexion are_____
    a. Inferior glide of patella, anterior glide of tibia and external rotation
    b. Inferior gliding of patella, posterior glide of tibia and internal rotation
    c. Superior gliding of patella, posterior glide of tibia and external rotation
    d. Superior gliding of patella, anterior glide of tibia and internal rotation
142. Stair climbing requires approximately knee flexion
    a. 85 degrees   b. 95 degrees
    c. 105 degrees   d. 115 degrees
143. Normal human locomotion requires _____ knee flexion
    a. 36 degrees   b. 67 degrees
    c. 98 degrees   d. 105 degrees
144. Meniscus injury occurs due to _____
    a. Valgus injury   b. Varus injury
    c. Dash board injury   d. Rotatory dysfunction
145. Dash board injury may give rise to _____
    a. Injury ACL   b. Injury MCL
    c. Injury PCL   d. Injury Meniscus

146. Squatting and descending the stairs become difficult in case of _____
    a. ACL injury
    b. PCL injury
    c. MCL injury
    d. Meniscus injury
147. Locking is a feature of _____ injury
    a. Collateral ligament
    b. Meniscus
    c. Cruciates
    d. All of the above
148. Hyperextension injury my result in tearing of _____
    a. Meniscus
    b. Collateral ligament
    c. ACL
    d. PCL
149. Running with turning and sharp cut is painful in _____ injury
    a. ACL,
    b. PCL
    c. Collateral ligament
    d. Meniscus
150. Haemarthrosis develops within _____ of injury and is very painful
    a. Minutes to hours
    b. Hours to days
    c. Days to weeks
    d. Weeks to months
151. Insidious onset of anterior/antero medial knee pain aggravated with activities involving knee bending is a feature of _____
    a. TF DJD
    b. PF DJD
    c. Ligamentous injury
    d. Meniscus injury.
152. Normal relation between the length of the patella and patellar tendon is _____
    a. Length of patella> patellar tendon
    b. Length of patellar tendon> patella
    c. Length of patellar tendon = patella
    d. No such relation exists
153. In patella alta _____
    a. Length of patellar tendon > patella
    b. Length of patella> patellar tendon
    c. Length of patellar tendon = patella
    d. None of the above
154. The Q angle is 13 to 18, it becomes 0 in _____.
    a. In lying with quadriceps contracting statically
    b. In high sitting with quadriceps relaxed

c. In high sitting with leg rotated externally
d. In standing with the quadriceps contracting statically

155. In high sitting with the legs hanging freely inferior pole of patella lies _____.
    a. Above the tibiofemoral joint line
    b. Below the tibiofemoral joint line
    c. At the level of tibiofemoral joint line
    d. None of the above

156. Positive valgus stress with the knee in extension indicates _____.
    a. Sprain MCL   b. Sprain ACL
    c. Sprain MCL &ACL   d. Sprain MCL with PCL.

157. In supine lying with knees bent at 60^0, less prominent tibial tubercle on one side indicates PCL rupture whereas more prominent tibial tubercle indicates_____.
    a. Rupture ACL
    b. Quadriceps contracture
    c. Patellofemoral tracking dysfunction
    d. Os Good schalter disease

158. You are evaluating a patient with injury to the posterior cruciate ligament. The mechanism of injury for the P.C.L is _____.
    a. Forceful landing on anterior tibia with knee hyper flexed.
    b. Anterior force on tibia when foot is fixed.
    c. Valgus force applied to knee when foot is fixed.
    d. Forced internal rotations of leg.

159. Positive apley's grinding test with external rotation of tibia and compression indicates lesion of _____.
    a. MCL   b. Medial Meniscus
    c. LCL   d. Lateral Meniscus

160. Quadriceps to hamstrings strength ration is _____.
    a. 2:1   b. 3:2
    c. 5:3   d. 5:4

161. During early phase of rehabilitation of ACL injury, managed conservatively or surgically, knee ROM is limited to _____
    a. 0 to 60   b. 10 to 90
    c. 45 to 90   d. Full range

162. For the rehabilitation of ACL emphasis should be given for the strengthening of _____ to regain stability
    a. Quadriceps
    b. Hamstrings
    c. Both quadriceps and hamstrings equally
    d. Quadriceps more than hamstrings
163. _____ is the recent trend for the management of meniscal injury
    a. Partial menisectomy
    b. Total menisectomy
    c. Meniscus repair
    d. Conservative treatment
164. A patient four weeks post arthroscopic menisectomy presents with knee flexion limitation. Which mobilization technique is beneficial to increase flexion ROM.
    a. Anterior glide of tibia
    b. Superior glide of patella
    c. posterior glide of tibia.
    d. Anterior glide fibular head
165. Following repair of anterior horn of medial meniscus ROM exercise is given by CPM, during which the hinge brace is locked between _____ range.
    a. 0 -90   b. 30 – 80
    c. 10 – 110   d. full
166. Following synovectomy ____.
    a. Immolisation is given till stitch removal
    b. Immolisation is given for 3 weeks
    c. Immolisation is given for 6 weeks
    d. Active movements can be initiated after 48-72 hours
167. The dynamic factors responsible to check lateral patellar tracking dysfunction is _____.
    a. Hip adduction   b. Vastus medialis
    c. Vastus lateralis   d. Rectus femoris
168. Surgical procedure for recurrent dislocation of patella is _____.
    a. Lateral retinacular release
    b. Medialisation of tibial tuberosity
    c. Vastus medialis transfer
    d. All of the above

169. Tibiofemoral compressive load increases with knee flexion because of _____
    a. Increase in weight transfer
    b. Increase in quadriceps contraction
    c. Increasing incongruence
    d. None
170. Patient with degenerative joint disease of knee joint presents with knee joint ROM of 20 to 100 degrees, complain of pain and difficulty in ADL. Which movement will you restore first?
    a. Flexion   b. Extension
    c. Both   d. None
171. Choose the correct statement regarding DJD.
    a. Loading the joint in incongruent positions predispose/precipitates DJD
    b. It manifests with capsular contracture and crepitus
    c. Capsular tightness predispose/precipitates DJD
    d. All of the above
172. Joint protection measures include _____.
    a. Reduction of body weight and avoidance of weight bearing activities
    b. Capsular stretching and muscle strengthening
    c. Use of orthosis for correct alignment of the joint and use of walking aids to reduce joint loading
    d. All of the above
173. Physiotherapy management for OA knee includes _____.
    a. Joint mobilization and stretching to correct deformities
    b. Small arc muscle endurance/strengthening to deload the joint
    c. Prophylactic measures and Proprioceptive training
    d. All of the above
174. Following cemented TKR, patient weans from crutches by _____.
    a. Stitch removal   b. 3 weeks
    c. 6 weeks   d. 3 months

175. Uncemented TKR patient can walk after_____.
    a. Stitch removal
    b. 3 weeks
    c. 6 weeks
    d. 3 months.
176. A patient post knee replacement is referred to you for ROM and strengthening exercise. Which treatment you my not choice for this patient.
    a. Active stretching by contract and relax
    b. Joint mobilization to gain joint play.
    c. SLR
    d. Closed kinetic chain exercise
177. The direction of displacement following supracondylar fracture femur is __
    a. Proximal fracture segment is displaced backward limiting flexion
    b. Proximal fracture segment is displaced forward limiting extension
    c. Distal fracture segment is displaced backward limiting extension
    d. Distal fracture segment is displaced forward limiting flexion
178. Clean cut fracture separation of patella is managed by _____.
    a. Conservatively
    b. Tension band wiring
    c. Patellectomy
    d. All of the above
179. A patient sustains fracture of the upper fibula with injury to the common peroneal nerve. Power of dorsifexors and evertors are 2/5. the most suitable management to help the patient with ADL is _____
    a. Electrical stimulation
    b. Orthosis
    c. Exercise programme
    d. Hydrotherapy
180. Deltoid ligament refers to _____
    a. MCL of ankle
    b. LCL of ankle
    c. Inferior tibiofibular ligament
    d. Talocalcaneal ligament
181. _____ is the most frequently injured ligament about the ankle
    a. Calcaneofibular ligament
    b. Deltoid ligament

c. Anterior talofibular ligament
d. Posterior talofibular ligament
182. Plantar calcaneo navicular ligament is referred as _____
    a. Interosseous ligament
    b. Spring ligament
    c. Deltoid ligament
    d. Bifurcate ligament
183. Anterior talofibular ligament checks _____
    a. Posterior movement of leg over talus, external rotation of leg and inversion
    b. Posterior movement of leg over talus, internal rotation of leg and inversion
    c. Anterior movement of leg over talus, internal rotation of leg and eversion
    d. Anterior movement of leg over talus, external rotation of leg and eversion
184. The mechanism of injury of anterior talofibular ligament is _____
    a. Eversion
    b. Inversion
    c. Combined plantar flexion and inversion
    d. Combination of dorsi flexion an diversion
185. In neutral standing with the feet pointed outward about 10, patella faces inward indicates _____
    a. Internal rotation of hip
    b. Internal rotation of leg
    c. Anteversion of femur
    d. Internal tibial torsion
186. Squinting patella with neutral hip rotation ROM indicates _____
    a. Internal rotation of hip
    b. Femoral retroversion
    c. External tibial torsion
    d. All
187. The component motion for ankle dorsiflexion is _____
    a. Anterior glide of talus in the mortise
    b. Posterior gliding of talus in the mortise

c. Compression of inferior tibiofibular joint
d. Inversion of talus
188. Foot pronation includes _____
   a. Plantar flexion, eversion adduction
   b. Plantar flexion, inversion, abduction
   c. Plantar flexion, inversion, adduction.
   d. Dorsiflexion, eversion, abduction
189. Supination of foot is the combination of_____
   a. Ankle DF subtalar eversion and forefoot abduction
   b. Ankle PF subtalar inversion and forefoot adduction
   c. Ankle DF subtalar inversion and forefoot abduction
   d. Ankle PF subtalar eversion and forefoot adduction
190. The axis of the ankle joint is directed backward and downward medio laterally, it makes about _____
   a. 25 from the frontal plane and 10 to 15 from transverse plane
   b. 25 from the obiliza plane and 10 to 15 from transverse plane
   c. 40 from the obiliza plane and 30 from transverse plane
   d. 40 from the frontal plane and 30 from transverse plane
191. When a ligament of the ankle completely torn the injury should be classified as
   a. Grade I sprain   b. Grade II sprain
   c. Grade III sprain   d. Grade IV sprain
192. Connective tissue disease tend to be disorder of _____.
   a. Males in 2nd decade
   b. Females after menopause
   c. Females in child bearing age
   d. Females in cold climatic conditions
193. A patient is said to have rheumatoid arthritis if he/she has at least _____ criteria out of seven
   a. 3   b. 4
   c. 5   d. All the seven
194. Haemosiderin deposit in synovium occurs in_____.
   a. Gout   b. Haemophilia
   c. Tabes dorsalis   d. Reiter's syndrome

195. Essence of pathology in RA is _____.
    a. Persistence synovitis
    b. Articular cartilage damage
    c. Deformities in joints
    d. Tendon ruptures
196. Enthesopathy occurs in _____.
    a. Rheumatoid arthritis
    b. Ankylosing spondylitis
    c. Psoriatic arthritis
    d. SLE
197. Lumbar spine is not involved in _____.
    a. Ankylosing spondylitis
    b. Rheumatoid arthritis
    c. Osteoarthritis
    d. None of the above
198. Enlarged spleen, lymphadenopathy anaemic with ulceration of legs is _____.
    a. Sjorgren's syndrome
    b. Reiter's syndrome
    c. Felty's syndrome
    d. Psoriatic arthritis
199. HLA B 27 is negative in _____.
    a. Ankylosing spondylitis
    b. Reiter's syndrome
    c. Psoriatic arthritis
    d. SLE
200. Neurological involvement in Rheumatoid arthritis includes ___.
    a. Compression of peripheral nerve due to tenosynovitis
    b. Peripheral neuropathy due to vasculitis
    c. SCI due to sulaxation/dislocation of atlanto-axial joint
    d. All of the above
201. Seronegative inflammatory arthritis conditions have a primary effect on _____.
    a. Axial skeleton
    b. Lumbar spine
    c. Big joints of the body
    d. Smaller joints of the body

202. Sausage fingers are found in_____.
   a. Rheumatoid arthritis
   b. Psoriatric arthritis
   c. Scleroderma
   d. Gout
203. Herberden's nodes are present in_____.
   a. Wrist
   b. Subcutaneous tissue
   c. DIP
   d. Shin of tibia
204. Sjogren's syndrome and felty's syndrome are variants of _____.
   a. SLE
   b. Scleroderma
   c. Rheumatoid arthritis
   d. Psoriatic arthritis
205. Serum uric acid level is higher in _____.
   a. SLE
   b. Stills disease
   c. Gout
   d. None of the above
206. Raynaud's phenomenon is the first presentation of_____.
   a. SLE
   b. Polymyositis
   c. Scleroderma
   d. Still's disease
207. Skin rash after exposure to sunlight is found in_____.
   a. Polymyositis
   b. SLE
   c. Scleroderma
   d. Gout
208. Modified New York criteria for the diagnosis of Ankylosing spondylosis includes_____.
   a. Insidious onset of morning stiffness and limited lumbar motion in two planes, improved by movements
   b. Bilateral Sacro-ilitis in X-rays
   c. Chest expansion less than 2.5 cm at nipple level
   d. All
209. Contractile tissue dysfunction is characterized by____.
   a. Pain during resisted isometric contraction and passive stretching
   b. Pain during passive movement
   c. Pain during joint play
   d. Pain during active movement

210. Noncontractile tissue dysfunction is characterized by ____.
    a. Pain during resisted isometric contraction
    b. Pain during active movement
    c. Pain during passive movement and joint play
    d. None of the above
211. Cyriax's DTFM for the ligament is given in _____
    a. Relaxed position followed by active movement
    b. Taut position followed by active movement
    c. Variable joint position followed by passive movement
    d. Any position followed by passive movement
212. Cyriax principle of management for spinal problems is _____
    a. Oscillatory rhythmic gliding
    b. Traction and manipulation
    c. Self treatment
    d. DTFM and injection
213. Adhesion within the muscle is characterized by
    a. Reduced active movement while passive ROM is full
    b. Reduction of passive ROM
    c. Reduced broadening of muscle/bulk during active contraction
    d. Pain during resisted isometric contraction
214. Adhesion of tendon with its sheath is characterized by _____
    a. Decreased of active movement while passive movement is full
    b. Decreased passive stretching
    c. Crepitus
    d. Pain during resisted isometric contraction
215. DTFM to the tendon is given with the _____
    a. Muscle is relaxed position
    b. Joint in variable positions
    c. Tendon is taut position
    d. Muscle in contracted position
216. Following DTFM to the muscle _____ should be encouraged.
    a. Active movement
    b. Passive stretching

c. Resisted movement
d. Active assisted movement
217. The rate of movement for DTFM is _____ cycles/sec
 a. 1-2 b. 2-3
 c. 3-4 d. 4-5
218. The effects of deep transverse friction massage includes____.
 a. It disperses the exudates and relieves pain
 b. Prevents/breaks adhesion
 c. Induces local erythema
 d. All of the above
219. McKenzie's derangement model is characterized by _____
 a. Repeated movement in the direction of derangement produces centralization of symptoms.
 b. Repeated movement in opposite direction of derangement produces centralization of symptoms.
 c. Repeated movement in the direction of derangement aggravates the symptoms.
 d. None of the above
220. According to Mckenzie, in case of derangement pain is relieved by _____
 a. Opening of IVF
 b. Pain gate theory
 c. Reduction of the deranged disc material
 d. Not known
221. McKenzie's dysfunction syndrome is characterized by _____
 a. Pain at end range, and restricted range of motion due to stretching of tight structure
 b. Repeated movement in the direction of dysfunction relieves the symptoms.
 c. Repeated movement in opposite direction of dysfunction aggravates the symptoms.
 d. None of the above

222. The treatment for McKenzie's dysfunction syndrome is
   a. Repeated movement in the direction of dysfunction movement
   b. Sustained movement in the opposite direction of dysfunction
   c. Posture correction
   d. Traction
223. McKenzie recommends for flexion exercises in case of posterior derangement syndrome
   a. Once patient remains pain free for 3 days
   b. Once patient remains pain free for 1 weeks
   c. Once patient remains pain free for 3 weeks
   d. Once patient remains pain free for 6 weeks
224. Ceralization of pain occurs in_____.
   a. Dysfunction   b. Derangement
   c. Postural syndrome   d. All of the above
225. Centralization is characterized by _____
   a. Shifting of pain to more proximal part over time
   b. Decrease of intensity of pain
   c. Decrease of duration of pain
   d. All of the above
226. Repetitive movement in the direction of derangement is recommended by McKenzie. The number of repetition should be _____
   a. 10-15   b. 15 – 20
   c. 20 – 30   d. 30 – 50
227. According to McKenzie treatment for unilateral/ asymmetrical pain with scoliosis deformity is____.
   a. First correct the listing
   b. Lay down in prone
   c. Spinal extension in prone
   d. Traction
228. Maitland's manual therapy concept is a clinical concept having two compartments, theoretical and clinical with a permeable wall in between. The core concept includes___.
   a. Subjective and objective evaluation
   b. Listen to the patient and believe him
   c. Formulate working hypothesis
   d. All of the above

229. Joint play is differentiated from physiological movement _____
    a. It occurs in anatomical planes
    b. It can be produced voluntarily
    c. It can be measured
    d. It can not be seen from outside
230. Joint gliding is defined as _____.
    a. The reference point on the movable surface comes in contact with variables points of the stationary surface
    b. The reference point on the movable surface comes in contact with a fixed point of the stationary surface
    c. The reference point on the movable surface comes in contact with variables points of the stationary surface at regular intervals
    d. None of the above
231. Joint rolling can be defined as _____.
    a. The reference point on the movable surface comes in contact with variables points of the stationary surface
    b. The reference point on the movable surface comes in contact with a fixed point of the stationary surface
    c. The reference point on the movable surface comes in contact with variables points of the stationary surface at regular intervals
    d. None of the above
232. Maitland's SIN group is characterized by _____.
    a. Pain encountered before motion barrier
    b. Pain encountered after motion barrier
    c. Pain and motion barrier encountered together
    d. None of the above
233. Maitland's Rhythmic oscillation mobilization technique can be applied_____.
    a. Only for joint play (Gliding)
    b. Only for physiological movement
    c. Both for joint play and physiological movement
    d. None
234. Lateral PA mobilization is applied on _____
    a. The painful side   b. Pain free side
    c. Both the sides   d. Either of side

235. Grade _____ mobilization is given for SIN group
   a. I b. II
   c. I and II d. III and IV
236. To improve JROM which grade mobilizations are used _____
   a. I and II b. II and III
   c. III and IV d. None of the above
237. Medium speed in maitland's mobilization is equal to _____
   a. ½ per sec b. 1 per sec
   c. 2 per sec d. 3 per sec
238. Transverse pressure on right side of spinous process _____
   a. Opens the foramen on left
   b. Closes the foramen on left
   c. Opens the foramen on right
   d. Opens on both the sides
239. For bilateral symptoms of the extremities of spinal origin ____ mobilization technique is recommended by Maitland.
   a. Central PA over spinous process
   b. Lateral PA over articular pillar on the more painful side
   c. Transverse gliding from the less painful side
   d. None of the above
240. When the concave surface moves over the convex _____
   a. Gliding and rolling occurs in the direction of movement
   b. Gliding occurs in the direction of movement & rolling in opposite direction
   c. Rolling occurs in the direction of movement and gliding in the opposite direction
   d. Gliding and rolling occur in the opposite direction to the movement
241. Kaltenborn's GI traction is _____
   a. Small amplitude distraction to nullify joint compression forces without any distraction.

    b. The slack is taken up and the surrounding tissue are not stretched
    c. The joint is distracted to increase the joint space
    d. None of the above
242. At rest joint is subjected to _____
    a. Joint cohesive force
    b. Muscle contraction force
    c. Atmospheric pressure
    d. All of the above
243. In close packed position _____
    a. Intracapsular space is greater
    b. Joint loading is maximum
    c. Joint is most stable
    d. Joint is incongruent
244. Resting position is a position, where the _____.
    a. Joint volume is maximum and pressure is minimum
    b. Capsuloligamentous structures are laxed
    c. Joint is incongruent and least stable
    d. All of the above
245. Injury in closed pack position results into_____.
    a. Fracture   b. Dislocation
    c. Sublaxation   d. Avulsion
246. _____ is the characteristic of muscle spasm.
    a. Limitation of active movement with pain
    b. Limitation of passive movement
    c. Limitation of joint play
    d. All of the above
247. The physiological motion barrier shifts towards the beginning and passive joint range of motion is restricted in case of _____ lesion.
    a. Muscle spasm   b. Ligamentous
    c. Bony   d. Skin
248. Anatomical barrier shifts to left in case of _____
    a. Muscle spasm
    b. Ligamentous shortening
    c. Bony restriction
    d. None of the above
249. The coupling movement in cervical spine is ___.
    a. Side flexion and rotation occur in the same direction

b. Side flexion and rotation occur in the opposite direction
c. Direction depends on cervical spine flexion/extension position
d. Side flexion and rotation occur independently

250. The coupling movement in thoracic spine is ___.
   a. Side flexion and rotation occur in the same direction
   b. Side flexion and rotation occur in the opposite direction
   c. Direction depends on cervical spine flexion/extension position
   d. Side flexion and rotation occur independently

251. The coupling movement in lumber spine is ___.
   a. Side flexion and rotation occur in the same direction
   b. Side flexion and rotation occur in the opposite direction
   c. Side flexion and rotation occur in the same direction when the spine is flexed and opposite direction when it is neutral or extended
   d. Side flexion and rotation occur independently

252. Creep is the characteristic property of viscoelastic structures, which is defined as____
   a. Elongation over time with the load remaining constant
   b. Load reduces over time with the length remaining constant
   c. Elongation is slower than recoil
   d. Relaxation is slower than lengthening

253. Choose the correct statement
   a. Tissue elongation is faster than relaxation
   b. Tissue elongation is slower than relaxation
   c. Rate of tissue elongation is equal to relaxation
   d. None of the above

254. Rate of tissue elongation is faster than relaxation because_____.
   a. Rate of fluid reabsorption is faster than rate of fluid release.
   b. Rate of fluid release is faster than rate of fluid reabsorption

c. Elongation is an active process, whereas relaxation is passive
d. Relaxation requires more energy than elongation

255. Mobilisation with movement concept was developed by ____.
   a. Mannel   b. Maitland
   c. Mulligan   d. Cyriax

256. Principle of Mulligan's manual therapy is _____.
   a. Self treatment technique
   b. Sustained gliding in the treatment plane
   c. Pain free active movement in weight bearing position is done, which is otherwise painful
   d. All of the above

257. The human spine has __ segments.
   a. 24   b. 29
   c. 33   d. 37

258. Total 23 presacral vertebrae indicate ____.
   a. Lumberisation of sacral vertebra
   b. Sacralisation of lumber vertebra
   c. Supernumery thoracic or lumbar vertebra
   d. None of the above

259. The thoracic kyphotic curve is due to ____.
   a. Wedge shaped IVD with lesser anterior height
   b. Wedge shaped vertebral body with lesser anterior height
   c. Wedge shaped vertebral body and IVD with lesser anterior height
   d. Wedge shaped vertebral body with lesser anterior height and wedge shaped IVD with greater anterior height

260. The cervical lordosis is due to ____.
   a. Wedge shaped IVD with greater anterior height
   b. Wedge shaped vertebral body with greater anterior height
   c. Wedge shaped vertebral body and IVD with lesser anterior height
   d. Wedge shaped vertebral body with greater anterior height and wedge shaped IVD with lesser anterior height

261. The spine has ___ motion segments.
    a. 23 b. 24
    c. 32 d. 34
262. The zygapophyseal joint can bear up to___ load depending on spinal posture.
    a. 10 – 25% b. 25 -33%
    c. 33 – 50% d. None of the above
263. The facets in the cervical region are oriented _____.
    a. 45 to frontal plane and parallel to transverse plane
    b. 45 to transverse plane and parallel to frontal plane
    c. 60 to transverse plane and 20 to frontal plane
    d. 45 to frontal plane and 90 to transverse plane
264. Lumbar facet joints are almost parallel to saggital plane allowing____.
    a. More of flexion-extension, less side flexion, but no rotation
    b. More rotation, less flexion-extension and no side flexion
    c. More side flexion, less flexion-extension, but no rotation
    d. More of flexion-extension, less rotation, but no side flexion
265. The disc space in young adults contributes to about _____ of total vertebral column height.
    a. 10-20% b. 20-33%
    c. 34-45% d. 46-50%
266. The intervertebral disc derives its nutrition _____
    a. Directly from the vessels supplying it
    b. From the synovial fluid
    c. From the vertebral bodies above and below it through the vertebral end plates
    d. From the surrounding tissues
267. Traction reduces the intra discal pressure, during the traction phase the disc absorb the fluid and the negative intra discal pressure gradually neutralizes over time. So
    a. Sustained traction should not be applied more than 10-12 minutes
    b. Release of sustained traction increases the intradiscal pressure and aggravates the symptoms

c. Intermittent traction can be applied for longer duration
   d. All of the above
268. PID is more common during____ years of age.
   a. 20-30   b. 30-40
   c. 40-50   d. Any age
269. Movement present at altanto-occipital joint are_____.
   a. Flexion-extension, some side flexion, but no rotation
   b. Rotation, some flexion-extension, but no side fiexion
   c. Side flexion , some flexion-extension, but no rotation
   d. Flexion-extension, some rotation and less side flexion
270. To check the movement of upper cervical spine, lock the lower cervical spine in full flexion.
   a. Movement of atlanto-occipital joint is tested by side flexion
   b. Movement of atlanto-axial joint is tested by side flexion
   c. Movement of atlanto-occipital joint is tested by rotation
   d. Movement of atlanto-occipital joint is tested by flexion-extension
271. Migraine must be excluded before treating cervical spine, which is characterized by___.
   a. Intermittent throbbing headache, blurring vision, nausea etc. related to activities
   b. Intermittent throbbing headache, blurring vision, nausea etc. unrelated to activities
   c. Intermittent throbbing headache, blurring vision, nausea etc. reproduced by rotation, extension and side flexion to painful side
   d. None of the above
272. Side flexion of head and neck to right includes___.
   a. Side flexion, rotation of lower cervical spine to right with slight extension and full rotation of atlant-axial joint to left, side flexion of atlanto-occipital joint to right in slight flexion
   b. Side flexion and rotation of cervical spine to right
   c. Side flexion to right and rotation left

    d. Side flexion to left and rotation of lower cervical spine to right with slight extension and full rotation of atlant-axial joint to left, side flexion of atlanto-occipital joint to right in slight flexion
273. Head forward posture may give rise to____.
    a. Flexion dysfunction of upper cervical spine and extension dysfunction of lower
    b. PID lower cervical spine/TOS
    c. Impingement syndrome/periarthritis
    d. All of the above
274. Flexion injury leading to anterior wedge fracture of vertebral body is common ___ region.
    a. Cervical   b. Thoracic
    c. Lumbar   d. Thoraco-lumbar
275. _____ injury of spine may lead to displacement and SCI.
    a. Flexion
    b. Hyperextension
    c. Flexion-rotation
    d. Vertical compression
276. The common site of fracture dislocation is TL region, which results from flexion-rotation injury. The method of management is___.
    a. Positional reduction by lying supine with pillow support
    b. Manipulative reduction
    c. ORIF
    d. Traction
277. Protrusion with complete rupture of annulus allowing the nucleus to bulge into the neural canal is referred as ____.
    a. Herniation
    b. Extrusion
    c. Sequestration
    d. Noncontained disc
278. The normal sequence of degeneration is ____.
    a. Annular tear, hypermobility, stabilization
    b. Hypermobility, annular tear, stabilization
    c. Stabilization, annular tear, hypermobility,
    d. None of the above

279. Which ligament in our body contains more elastin fibres?
    a. Longitudinal ligament
    b. Interspinous ligament
    c. Ligamentum nuchae
    d. Ligamentum flavum
280. Locked facet in the lumbar spine is due to ____.
    a. Localized hypermobility
    b. Failure of ligamentum flavum
    c. Muscle weakness
    d. Unguarded movements
281. Posterolateral disc prolapse in lumbar spine is common, why?
    a. Disc lies more posteriorly
    b. Load is more
    c. Posterior longitudinal ligament is narrower
    d. All of the above
282. About 90-95% persons with PID lists away from the painful side, while rest of 5-10% lists towards the same side indicating prolapse medial to the root, which is characterized by____.
    a. Side flexion towards the sound side aggravates the symptoms
    b. Lateral PA pressure over sound side reproduces the symptoms
    c. Traction aggravates the symptoms
    d. All of the above
283. Choose the correct statement regarding intradiscal pressure.
    a. IDP in semifowler position > supine
    b. IDP in supine > side lying
    c. IDP in lying > standing
    d. IDP in sitting > standing
284. Sequence of physiotherapy for PID are_____.
    a. Passive mobilization, traction, stretching, auto assisted exercise, active exercises
    b. Traction, stretching, mobilization, active exercises, assisted exercise
    c. Active exercises, auto assisted exercise, stretching, traction, mobilization

d. Autoassisted exercise, active exercises, mobilization, stretching, traction
285. Spondylosis is characterized by ____.
    a. Hypermobility   b. Stiff spine
    c. Spinal instability   d. Locking
286. Physiotherapy management of Spondylolisthesis excludes____.
    a. Back extension exercises
    b. Stretching of hip flexors, hamstrings
    c. Spinal flexion exercises
    d. Spinal stabilisation exercise
287. When treating an acute lumbo – strain the treatment choice is _____
    a. Hot packs and ultra sound
    b. Extension exercises
    c. Flexion exercises
    d. Difficult to decide based on information given
288. All of the following are true concerning scoliosis except _____
    a. A 15 degree to 20 degree curve is mild curve
    b. Bracing is an effective treatment tool
    c. Scoliosis is named by the direction of concavity
    d. Early detection is essential.
289. The most common cause for lower limb amputations is _____.
    a. Congenital deformities
    b. Infection
    c. Trauma
    d. Vascular disease
290. Stitching opposite group of muscles with each other to cover the distal end of the stump is known as ____ technique of amputation.
    a. Myodesis   b. Myoplasty
    c. Closed   d. Open
291. The purpose of stump bandaging includes all of the following except _____
    a. Provides protection against accidental injuries
    b. Reduces edema

c. Supports for surgical wound
d. Prevents contractures
292. Physiotherapy for phantom pain or phantom limb sensation includes TENS. Where will you place the electrodes?
    a. Stump end
    b. One over the painful site and other over the nerve trunk
    c. One over the stump end and other over the dermatome
    d. Any where over the stump
293. Active stump exercises can be started after____.
    a. Removal of the drainage tube
    b. Stitch removal
    c. 3 weeks
    d. 6 weeks
294. In case of AK amputee prosthetic knee stabilization can be achieved by____.
    a. Action of gluteus maximus
    b. Trochanteric knee alignment
    c. Extension aid
    d. All of the above
295. Neurovascular deficits are common complications of fracture____ of femur.
    a. Shaft
    b. Supracondylar
    c. Trochanter
    d. Condyles
296. Haemophilics should avoid____.
    a. IM injection
    b. Contact games
    c. Intake of Aspirin and other NSAID
    d. All of the above
297. Physiotherapy after bleeding in haemophilic can be started ____.
    a. Once bleeding stops, characterized by reduction of swelling, pain and warmth
    b. Within 8 – 24 hours of factor infusion
    c. Once isometric contraction of the overlying muscle is possible
    d. All of the above

298. Physiotherapy in haemophilia includes ___.
   a. Ice and rest following acute bleeding
   b. Early isometric contractions followed by active exercises to strengthen muscles
   c. Gradual stretching and joint mobilization with the traction
   d. All of the above
299. Therapeutic modality used in haemophilia ___.
   a. US   b. PEME
   c. IFT/ES   d. All of the above
300. Charcoat joints are ___.
   a. Painless arthritic joint disease
   b. Degeneratine joint disease
   c. Infective joint disease
   d. Ankylosed joints

ANSWER SHEET OF PT IN ORTHOPADIC CONDITIONS

1. a	2. b	3. c	4. a	5. b
6. a	7. d	8. d	9. b	10. a
11. c	12. a	13. b	14. c	15. b
16. a	17. a	18. a	19. b	20. c
21. b	22. b	23. c	24. c	25. b
26. c	27. b	28. d	29. b	30. b
31. a	32. b	33. d	34. d	35. b
36. b	37. b	38. a	39. d	40. a
41. c	42. b	43. a	44. a	45. b
46. a	47. d	48. b	49. d	50. b
51. a	52. c	53. b	54. b	55. b
56. d	57. b	58. b	59. b	60. b
61. b	62. a	63. d	64. b	65. b
66. a	67. b	68. b	69. c	70. b
71. c	72. a	73. b	74. b	75. b
76. c	77. c	78. a	79. c	80. c
81. d	82. b	83. b	84. c	85. d
86. a	87. a	88. b	89. a	90. c
91. d	92. b	93. b	94. c	95. c
96. a	97. b	98. a	99. a	100. c
101. b	102. c	103. a	104. c	105. b
106. d	107. b	108. c	109. b	110. b
111. d	112. d	113. a	114. b	115. c
116. d	117. d	118. a	119. d	120. d

121. d	122. d	123. b	124. c	125. a
126. d	127. b	128. a	129. a	130. a
131. c	132. c	133. a	134. a	135. a
136. a	137. b	138. d	139. a	140. a
141. b	142. a	143. b	144. d	145. c
146. b	147. b	148. d	149. c	150. a
151. b	152. c	153. a	154. b	155. c
156. c	157. d	158. a	159. b	160. b
161. c	162. b	163. c	164. c	165. b
166. d	167. b	168. d	169. c	170. b
171. d	172. d	173. d	174. c	175. b
176. b	177. c	178. b	179. b	180. a
181. c	182. b	183. a	184. c	185. c
186. c	187. b	188. d	189. b	190. a
191. c	192. c	193. b	194. b	195. a
196. b	197. b	198. b	199. d	200. d
201. a	202. b	203. c	204. c	205. c
206. c	207. a	208. d	209. a	210. c
211. c	212. b	213. c	214. a	215. c
216. a	217. b	218. d	219. a	220. c
221. a	222. b	223. a	224. b	225. d
226. a	227. a	228. d	229. d	230. a
231. c	232. a	233. c	234. a	235. c
236. c	237. b	238. a	239. a	240. a
241. a	242. d	243. c	244. d	245. a
246. d	247. b	248. c	249. a	250. b
251. c	252. a	253. a	254. b	255. c
256. d	257. c	258. b	259. b	260. a
261. a	262. b	263. b	264. a	265. b
266. c	267. c	268. b	269. a	270. a
271. b	272. a	273. d	274. b	275. c
276. a	277. b	278. a	279. b	280. b
281. d	282. d	283. c	284. b	285. b
286. a	287. d	288. c	289. c	290. b
291. d	292. b	293. b	294. d	295. a
296. d	297. d	298. d	299. d	300. a

CHAPTER 4

Physiotherapy in Neurological Conditions

1. Erb's palsy affects
   a. Lumbar plexus   b. Sacral plexus
   c. Brachial plexus   d. Cranial nerves.
2. Pain sensation is carried by
   a. Medial spinothalamic tract
   b. Lateral spinothalamic tract
   c. Posterior column
   d. Anterior column
   3. Proprioceptive sensation ascend in spinal cord through_____ column
   a. Posterior
   b. Lateral
   c. Anterior
   d. Anterolateral
4. Boca's area of brain is for
   a. Speech   b. Hearing
   c. Locomotion   d. Vision
5. Bell's palsy occurs when the injury is
   a. Above pons
   b. At the pons

c. At zygomastoid foramen
   d. None of the above
 6. Dorsal spinocerebellar tract relays afferent information from muscle spindles from which part of body?
   a. Upper region   b. Lower region
   c. Trunk   d. None of the above.
 7. Which lesion of motor cortex has poorest prognosis?
   a. Primary cortex   b. Premotor cortex
   c. Internal capsule d. Supplementary motor cortex.
 8. Primary motor cotex area 4 lesion causes paralysis of____.
   a. Contralateral spastic paralysis upper limb
   b. Ipsilateral spastic paralysis lower limb
   c. Contralateral upper limb, upper limb, face.
   d. None of the above
 9. Premotor area (area 6) lesion result in_____.
   a. Slowing of movement
   b. Hypertonia
   c. Inability to develop appropriate movement
   d. a and c
10. Appreciation of localization of light touch is lost when there is injury of_____.
    a. Thalamus   b. Brainstem
    b. Sensory cortex c. Peripheral nerve
11. Supplemental motor area lesion will result in_____.
    a. Motor apraxia in the absence of motor or sensory impairment
    b. Spastic paralysis contralateral
    c. Flaccid paralysis of ipsilateral
    d. In co-ordination
12. Decusation of corticospinal tract occur at _____.
    a. Spinal cord
    b. Junction of medulla and spinal cord
    c. Above medulla
    d. Pons
13. Dopamine is synthesized by_____.
    a. Globus pallidum
    b. Substantia nigra

c. Subthalmaic nucleus
   d. Putamen
14. Paleocerebellum chiefly concerned with_____.
    a. Information from stretch receptors.
    b. Voluntary function
    c. Involuntary function
    d. Posture
15. Which somatosensory system possess more discriminative properties?
    a. Spinothlamic   b. Lemniseal
    c. Spinocerebellar   d. None of the above
16. Merkel's disk is responsible for _____ sensation.
    a. Touch – pressure
    b. Touch temperature
    c. Two point discrimination
    d. Stereognosis
17. Meissner's corpuscle is responsible for_____ sensation.
    a. Two point discrimination steriognosis
    b. Touch
    c. Temperature
    d. Pressure
18. Cortical sensation is mediated by_____.
    a. Primary somatosensory area
    b. Skin receptors
    c. Secondary somatosensory cortex
    d. Secondary somatosensory cortex and posterior multimodal association area
19. Motor planning and timing take place by lobe of cerebellum.
    a. Anterior lobe   b. Floculonodular
    c. Posterior   d. All of the above
20. Ventral spinocerebellar signals from tracts carry
    a. Lower limb   b. Upper limb
    c. Trunk   d. a and b
21. Short term memory is mediated by_____.
    a. Limbic system   b. Frontal lobe
    c. Hippo campus   d. Parietal lobe

22. In two point discrimination the distance between two points in palm is_____.
    a. 5 – 6 mm   b. 7 – 10 mm
    c. 10- 15 mm   d. None
23. Short term memory is mediated by_____.
    a. Limbic system   b. Frontal lobe
    c. Hippo campus   d. Parietal lobe
24. Cortical sensation is mediated by_____.
    a. Primary somato sensory area
    b. Skin receptors
    c. Secondary somato sensory cortex
    d. Secondary somatosensory cortex and posterior multimodal association area
25. Patients with spinocerebellar tract lesion will lack_____.
    a. Ipsilateral upper limb control
    b. Ipsilateral upper limb and trunk control
    c. Ipsilateral lower limb & trunk control
    d. Contralateral upper limb and lower limb control.
26. Anterior cerebral artery lesion will result in_____.
    a. Ipsilateral lower limb sensory loss
    b. Ipsilateral upper limb sensory loss
    c. Contralateral lower limb sensory loss
    d. Both upper limb and lower limb sensory loss
27. Middle cerebral artery lesion will result in_____.
    a. Ipsilateral sensory loss of whole trunk
    b. Contralateral sensory loss of upper limb, lower limb and face
    c. Contralateral sensory loss of upper limb.
    d. None
28. Patients with subcortical lesion will have loss of sensation of _____.
    a. Contralateral upper limb.
    b. Contralateral upper limb and lower limb contralateral
    c. Contralateral upper limb, lower limb and face
    d. Ipsilateral upper limb, lower limb, trunk and face
29. Parietal lobe lesion exhibit_____.
    a. Lack of sensory motor integration
    b. Inability to interpret meaningful sensory information

c. Both a and b.
d. None
30. Facilitation of extensor tone against gravity occurs by _____.
    a. Vestibulo spinal tract
    b. Rubro spinal tract
    c. Reticulo spinal tract
    d. Corticospinal tract
31. Spastic diplegia is characterized by _____.
    a. Increased stiffness in both lower extremities, minimal involvement of upper extremities and trunk
    b. Increased stiffness in both upper extremities, minimal involvement of lower extremities and trunk
    c. Increased stiffness in one half of the body and minimal involvement of other half
    d. Increased stiffness in both lower extremities and trunk, but no involvement of upper extremities
32. Apraxia is a result of lesion in _____.
    a. Frontal lobe   b. Parietal lobe
    c. Occipital lobe   d. Internal capsule
33. Broca's area is present in_____.
    a. Frontal lobe   b. Parietal lobe
    c. Occipital lobe   d. Frontal lobe
34. _____nervous system is/are responsible for bladder evacuation.
    a. Sympathetic
    b. Parasympathetic
    c. Sympathetic and parasympathetic
    omatic
35. Deep tendon reflex is exaggerated in lesion_____.
    a. Upper motor neuron
    b. Lower motor neuron
    c. Peripheral nerve injury
    d. None of the above
36. Clonus is a sign of _____.
    a. Lower motor neuron lesion
    b. Upper motor neuron lesion
    c. Peripheral nerve injury
    d. All of the above.

37. Bilateral hemiplegia is characterized by _____.
    a. Increased stiffness in both lower extremities, minimal involvement of upper extremities and trunk
    b. Increased stiffness in both upper extremities, minimal involvement of lower extremities and trunk, but one half of the body is more involved than the other half
    c. Increased stiffness in both lower extremities and trunk, but no involvement of upper extremities
    d. None of the above
38. Which is dependant on velocity?
    a. Flaccidity
    b. Spasticity
    c. Rigidity
    d. None of the above
39. Loss of light touch sensation is ———.
    a. Atothiguranethesia
    b. Dysethesia
    c. Anesthesia
    d. Aptopogrosia
40. Removal of somatosensory (SII) area leads to ——
    a. Impairment of postural sense
    b. Impairment of perception of shape of object
    c. Impairment of perception of both shape & texture of object
    d. Impairment of perception of texture
41. Stroking across lateral border of foot elicits _____ reflex.
    a. Chaddock   b. Gordon
    c. Oppeneim   d. Babinski
42. Involuntary ballistic movement are due to the lesion of _____.
    a. Putamen
    b. Red nucleus
    c. Caudate nucleus
    d. Subthalamic nuclei
43. Meralgia parasthetica occurs in_____ nerve.
    a. Sciatic
    b. Superficial peroneal

c. Lateral femoral cutaneous
   d. Sural
44. Decerebrate rigidity refers to _____.
   a. Sustained contraction and posturing of the trunk and limbs in a position of full flexion
   b. Sustained contraction and positioning of the trunk and limbs in a position of full extension
   c. Sustained contraction and posturing of the trunk and the lower limbs in extension and the upper limbs in flexion
   d. Strong and sustained contraction of extensors muscles of the neck, trunk and four limbs
45. Thermanalgesia is _____.
   a. Inability to perceive heat
   b. Inability to perceive sensation of heat and cold
   c. Inability to perceive pain and temperature
   d. None of the above.
46. Features of diabetic neuropathy
   a. Mild and chronic
   b. b. Affecting both sensory and motor nerve
   c. Lower extremity involvement
   d. b and c
   e. a , b and c
47. The differentiating feature of diabetes from tabes is _____.
   a. Pain
   b. Ataxia
   c. Loss of tendon reflex in lower limb
   d. Tender calf
48. The differentiating feature of poly neuropathy from polio myelitis is _____.
   a. Muscle weakness
   b. Muscle atrophy
   c. No sensory involvement
   d. Symmetrical muscle involvement
49. Which is not a feature of myasthenia gravis?
   a. Muscle weakness
   b. Muscle wasting

c. Muscle fatigability
d. Fasciculation
50. MND involves progressive degeneration of _____.
    a. Anterior horn cells of in the spinal cord
    b. Cells of lower cranial motor nuclei
    c. Neurons of the motor cortex and pyramidal tract
    d. All of the above
51. Parietal cerebral tumor cause_____.
    a. Progressive dementia
    b. Contralateral hemiplegia
    c. Falling away of contra lateral outstretched hand
    d. Epilepsy with aphasia
52. Apraxia is a result of lesion in _____.
    a. Frontal lobe   b. Parietal lobe
    c. Occipital lobe   d. Internal capsule
53. An uniform resistance at all points of range during relaxed passive movement is known as _____ spasticity.
    a. Clasp knife   b. Lead pipe
    c. Cog wheel   d. All of the above
54. The physiological basis of spasticity is_____.
    a. Increased fusimotor innervation by dynamic gamma motor neuron
    b. Decreased presynaptic inhibition
    c. Loss of reciprocal innervation and recurrent inhibition
    d. a and b
    e. a, b and c
55. The dyskinesia which resembles fragments of purposive movement is_____.
    a. Dystonia   b. Chorea
    c. Hemiballismus   d. Athetosis
56. Fasciculation is not found in_____.
    a. Cervical myelopathy
    b. Syringomyelia
    c. Stroke
    d. Intervertibral disc protrusion
57. A cerebral cortical lesion usually causes_____.
    a. Monoplegia   b. Hemiplegia
    c. Quadriplegia   d. Crossed hemiplegia

58. Which one among the following is true for polyneuropathy?
    a. Asymmetrical loss of reflex
    b. Distal tendon reflexes affected before proximal
    c. All reflexes are diminished
    d. All reflexes are lost
59. Oppenheim's reflex is_____.
    a. Extension of great toe with firm moving pressure on the skin over tibia
    b. Stroking on inner border elicits flexor respons
    c. Stroking outer border of sole elicits ankle dorsi flexion
    d. None of the above
60. Dissosiated sensory loss is found in_____.
    a. Polyneuropathy
    b. Lateral spinalcord lesion
    c. Central spinal cord lesion
    d. Spinothalamic tract lesion
61. The spinal segment for ankle jerk is_____.
    a. L5   b. L5S1
    c. S1S2   d. S1
62. Horner's syndrome is associated with_____.
    a. Myositis   b. Anhydrosis
    c. All of them   d. None of them
63. What happens in writer's cramp ?
    a. An act is impaired
    b. Individual movements which compose the act are impaired
    c. Similar activities are affected
    d. Associated with sensory loss
64. Transient ischemic attack usually defined if neurological deficit recovers with in _____.
    a. 24 hours   b. 48 hours
    c. > 24 hours< 7days. d. > 7 days.
65. The features of CSF leak is _____.
    a. fluid test positive for glucose
    b. salty taste in the mouth of the patient.
    c. There may be a fracture petrous skull
    d. All of the above
    e. a and c

66. Dysdiadokokinesia is a feature of _____.
    a. Basal ganglia lesion
    b. Cerebellar lesion
    c. Cortical lesion
    d. None of the above
67. Chorea is due to involvement of _____.
    a. Subthalamic nucleus
    b. Caudate and putamen
    c. Substantia nigra
    d. Basal ganglia
68. Worm like involuntary movement is _____.
    a. Chorea   b. Dystonia
    c. Athetosis   d. Hemiballismus
69. Lesion in one optic tract prouduce _____.
    a. Central scotoma
    b. Homonimous hemianopia
    c. Bi temporal hemianopia
    d. Blindness
70. The hallmark of space occupying lesion in brain are _____.
    a. Papilloedema   b. Headache
    c. Vomiting   d. b and c
    e. a b, and c
71. Sixth nerve palsy can cause_____.
    a. Squint   b. Diplopia
    c. Blindness   d. Ptosis
72. Rythmic oscillation of the eye is_____.
    a. Strabismus   b. Opthalmoplegia
    c. Nystagmus   d. None of the above
73. Emotional movement spaired with lower part of the face more affected when 7th cranial nerve is injured at_____.
    a. Pons
    b. Above pons
    c. Cerebellopontine angle
    d. Facial canal
74. Crocodile tear is feature of_____ cranial nerve palsy.
    a. 2nd   b. 3rd
    c. 6th   d. 7th

75. Which type of current is used usually in Bell's palsy?
    a. Faradic type   b. Interrupted galvanic
    c. Russian   d. Tens
76. Climbing up stairs need adequate_____.
    a. Gluteus maximus power in stable limb
    b. Abductor power in advancing limb
    c. Gluteus maximus and glueus medius power in stable limb
    d. Gluteus maximum and gluetus medius power in advancing limb
77. The first superficial reflex to recover following SCI is _____.
    a. Bulbocavernous   b. Anal
    c. Cremastric   d. Abdominal
78. Crede maneuver is used when there is _____.
    a. Automatic bladder
    b. Autonomous bladder
    b. Detrusor sphincter
    c. Flacid sphincter and spastic detrusor
79. The rhythm of tremor observed in Parkinson's disease at rest is about_____.
    a. 4-7 beats/second   b. 10-20 beats/second
    c. 4-7 beats/minute   d. 10-20 beats/minute
80. Pathological fixation of spinal cord in an abnormal caudal location is known as _____.
    a. Congenital fixation of spinal cord
    b. Fibrosis of spinal cord
    c. Diastometomyelia
    d. Tethered cord
81. Which is not feature of cerebellar dysfunction?
    a. Bradykinesia   b. Dysmetria
    c. Asthenia   d. Hypotonia
82. An uncomfortable hypersensitivity to non noxious stimuli is _____.
    a. Parasthesia   b. Hyperesthesia
    c. Disesthesia   d. None of the above
83. For two point discrimination on the trunk the distance between two points should be _____.

    a. 3 to 4 mm apart   b. 5 to 10 mm apart
    c. 10 to 20 mm apart   d. >30 mm apart
84. Babinski sign normally present up to age _____.
    a. Age 5 to 10   b. Age 10 to 15
    c. Age 1 to 2   d. Up to 6 months
85. Pain is uncommon in _____.
    a. Conus lesion
    b. Cauda equina lesion
    c. Higher thoracic lesion
    d. None of the above
86. There are how many grades in modified Ashworth scale for spasticiy?
    a. 3   b. 4
    c. 5   d. 6
87. What is normal grading of reflex?
    a. +   b. ++
    c. +++   d. —
88. Strabismus is _____.
    a. Ocular muscle imbalance and weakness
    b. Optic nerve damage
    c. Abnormal puple only constriction
    d. None
89. For near visual acquity the visual acuity chart is kept_____ away.
    a. 26"   b. 16"
    c. 10"   d. 40"
90. The distance for using snellen's chart is ————.
    a. Patient is 10 feet away
    b. Patient is 20 feet away
    c. Patient is 15 feet away
    d. None
91. Prosopagnosia is _____.
    a. Inability to recognize familiar objects
    b. Inability to identify familiar faces
    c. Inability to interpret visual stimuli
    d. Inability to remember appropriate colour
92. Astereognosis is indicated if patient is unable to identify_____ objects.

a. 2 or more
   b. 5 or more
   c. 3 or more
   d. 10 or more
93. Ability to interpret letter written on the palmar surface of one's hand is _____.
   a. Stereognosia   b. Ahylognosia
   c. Graphesthesia   d. None
94. Loss of hearing for low pitched tones is a feature of_____.
   a. Middle ear infection
   b. Damage of sensory end organ
   c. Damage of cochlear part of 8th nerve
   d. Auditory cortical area
95. Semicircular canals are excited by _____.
   a. Linear movement
   b. Angular movement
   c. Acceleration
   d. Decelleration
96. Vertigo means a feeling of _____.
   a. External world appear to move in arotatory fashion.
   b. External world oscillates
   c. Patient feels his own body moves/rotates
   d. a and b
   e. a, b and c
97. Which of the following is not a brain stem reflex?
   a. STNR   b. ATNR
   c. Positive supporting   d. Crossed extension
98. Modified ashworth scale grade 1+ _____
   a. Slight increase in muscle tone, manifested by a catch, followed by minimal resistance throughout the reminder (less than half) of the range of motion.
   b. Slight increase and tone, manifested by a catch and release and by minimal resistance at the end of the range when the affected part is moved in flexion and extension.
   c. More marked increase in tone, but affected part easily flexed
   d. Consideration increase in tone, passive movement difficult

99. The prognosis of meningitis depends upon _____.
    a. Infecting organism
    b. Stage of illness
    c. Presence of fracture skull
    d. All of the above
    e. a and b
100. Trigeminal neuralgia is caused by demyelinatio/degeneration of_____.
    a. Sensory divison of cranial nerve 5
    b. Motor division of cranial nerve 5.
    c. Sensory division of cranial nerve 6
    d .Motor division of cranial nerve 6
101. Commonest intra cranial tumor is _____.
    a. Gliomas   b. Meningiomas
    c. Angiomas   d. Neuromas
102. The example of operant/instrumental learning is ___.
    a. Assisted exercise with verbal command
    b. Constant repeated practice of a task
    c. Verbal praise after a well done task
    d. Non of the above
103. Learning task without attention is referred as _____.
    a. Classic condition
    b. Trail and error learning
    c. Instrumental learning
    d. Procedural learning
104. Declarative learning requires____.
    a. Repetition   b. Attention
    c. Reward   d. Assistance
105. Backer type of muscular dystrophy is_____.
    a. X-linked dominant
    b. Autosomal recessive
    c. None of them
    d. all of them
106. Charcots's joint is found in _____.
    a. Syringomyelia   b. Tabes dorsalis
    c. Diabetes myelitis   d. All of the above
    e. a and b
107. Which one of the following is known as Bell's palsy?
    a. 5th Cranial nerve palsy

b. 6th cranial nerve palsy
   c. 7th cranial nerve palsy
   d. None of the above
108. In poliomyelitis destruction occurs in _____.
   a. Muscle
   b. Peripheral nerve
   c. Anterior horn cells
   d. Posterior horn cells
109. Therapeutic modalities that reduce spasticity effectively_____.
   a. Ice
   b. Weight bearing
   c. Sustained stretching
   d. All of the above.
110. Spinal muscular atrophy type 4 and 5 presents_____.
   a. At infancy
   b. Childhood
   c. Pre pubescent
   d. After adolescence
111. Polymyositis is _____.
   a. Infective myopathy
   b. Inflammatory myopathy
   c. Not myopathy
   d. Muscle degenerating disease
112. Which one among the following is milder variety of neuromuscular disease?
   a. DMD
   b. BMD
   c. SMA type 1
   d. SMA type 2
113. Segmental demyelination is the predominant pathology in_____.
   a. Ischemic neuropathy
   b. Nutritional neuropathy
   c. Lead poisoning
   d. Guillain-bare syndrome
114. The chest wall mobility of parkinson's disease can be improved by using _____.
   a. PNF upper extremity bilateral symmetrical D2 flexion and extension   ans:a
   b. PNF upper extremity bilateral symmetrical D1 flexion and extension
   c. PNF one upper limb D12 flexion and extension and another upper limb D2 flexion and extension and vice versa.
   d. PNF one upper limb D2 flexion and extension with lower limb D2 flexion and extension and vice versa.

115. Weber's syndrome is _____.
    a. Occulomotor nerve palsy and contralateral hemiplegia
    b. Facial nerve palsy and contralateral hemiplegia
    c. Facial nerve, trigeminal nerve palsy and contralateral hemiplegia.
    d. Occulomotor abducens and optic nerve palsy and contralateral hemiplegia.
116. Wilson's disease is_____.
    a. Hepato lenticular degeneration
    b. Caused by disturbance of copper metabolism
    c. Frequently familial
    d. All of them
    e. a and b
117. Which one of the following technique is used in cerebellar ataxia?
    a. Rhythmic initiation
    b. Rhythmic stabilization
    c. Repeated contraction
    d. None of the above
118. Which is not related to favorable prognosis for patient with multiple sclerosis?
    a. Onset with only one symptoms.
    b. Relapsing – remitting variety
    c. Onset before the age of 40.
    d. Significant pyramidal and cerebellar signs with involvement at multiple sites in 5 years.
119. The disease nadir for Gullian Barre Syndrome should be within _____.
    a. 2 – 4 weeks   b. 2 months
    c. One week   d. 4 months
120. Body scheme perceptive disorders occur in _____.
    a. Left hemisphere lesion in posterior multi modal association area
    b. Right hemisphere lesion in posterior multi modal association area
    c. Left hemisphere anterior part
    d. Right anterior part

121. Arnold chiari malformation is associated with _____.
    a. Multiple sclerosis   b. Spina bifida
    c. Syringomyelia   d. b and c
122. Cervical rigidity, head retraction, kernig's sign are feature of _____.
    a. Encephalomyelitis   b. Cerebral abscess
    c. Meningitis   d. None of the above
123. Post-traumatic amnesia and retrograde amnesia are the features of _____.
    a. Cerebral contusion   b. Concussion
    c. Cerebral laceration   d. Cerebral compression
124. Paralysis of palate, pharynx and larynx can occur due to lesion of_____.
    a. 7th cranial nerve   b. 9th cranial nerve
    c. 10th cranial nerve   d. 12th cranial nerve
125. The ————— lesion will not produce hypotonia.
    a. Cerebellum   b. Reticular formation
    c. Anterior horn cell   d. Substantia nigra
126. The afferent side of spinal reflex arc is affected due to _____.
    a. Polyneuritis
    b. Peripheral nerve injury
    c. Tabes dorsalis
    d. Poliomyelitis
127. Language perception disorder is_____.
    a. Alexia   b. Aphasia
    c. Dyslexia   d. Broca's aphasia
128. Motor perception disorder is _____.
    a. Aphasia   b. Apraxia
    c. Alexia   d. Anomia
129. Friedreich's ataxia is due to a defect in chromosome _____.
    a. 9   b. 10
    c. 12   d. None
130. Which of the disease improves significantly with dopaminergic medications?
    a. Friedreich's ataxia
    b. Huntington's disease

c. Parkinson's disease
d. None

131. An increase of 5gm/l or higher in the protein content of CSF may be due to _____.
    a. Meningitis   b. Encephalytis
    c. Poliomyelitis   d. Acute infective polyneuritis

132. An increase in IgG fraction of gamma globulin with a normal total protein content is suggestive of _____.
    a. Polyneuropathy
    b. Meningitis
    c. Systemic lupus erythematosis
    d. Multiple sclerosis

133. Sub acute combined cord degeneration is due to _____.
    a. Vitamin B deficiency
    b. Vitamin B6 deficiency
    c. Vitamin B12 deficiency
    d. Vitamin B2 deficiency

134. Myelomeningocoele is a _____.
    a. Swelling containing meninges and CSF
    b. Swelling containing myelin sheath, meninges and CSF fluid
    c. Swelling containing spinal cord, meningocoele and CSF Fluid
    d. None of the above

135. Crossed hemiplegia means _____.
    a. Lesion above pontine
    b. At level of the pontine
    c. Below pontine
    d. None of the above.

136. Cerebral irritation may occur in _____.
    a. Concussion
    b. Moderate contusion
    c. Severe contusion
    d. Cerebral compression

137. In flexion and extension the length of the spinal canal varies from _____.
    a. 5 – 9 cm   b. 15 – 20 cm
    c. 10 – 20 cm   d. None of the above.

138. The blood supply to nerve fibers stops at _____ of elongation.
    a. 15% b. 5%
    c. 10% d. None of the above
139. Lines of pain and clumps of pain relates to involvement of _____.
    a. Muscle b. Nerve
    c. Joint d. Ligament
140. The resting membrane potential varies from _____ MV for most nerves, muscles and glial cells.
    a. – 40 to – 90 b. – 10 to – 100
    c. – 50 to + 90 d. – 40 to + 90
141. Symptoms worst at end of the day related to _____.
    a. Acute nerve root involvement
    b. Chronic Nerve Root Irritation
    c. Muscle ischemia
    d. None of the above.
142. Crossed SLR is said to be positive when with unilateral leg pain _____-
    a. the SLR on symptomatic leg side produces opposite limb symptom
    b. SLR on the sound side produces symptomatic leg's symptoms.
    c. SLR on both the sides are painful
    d. None of the above
143. The number of spinal nerves that emerge from spinal cord is _____.
    a. 33 pairs b. 31 pairs
    c. 32 pairs d. None of the above.
144. C1 dermatome is not there because _____.
    a. Dorsal root absent in cervical region
    b. Relation of spinal root with vertebral column
    c. C1 nerve root is absent
    d. C1 dorsal root supply inside the skull.
    e. None of the above.
145. The most common nerve used for biopsy in poly neuropathy is _____.
    a. Sural nerve b. Radial nerve

    c. Median nerve   d. Lateral cutaneous nerve of thigh

146. In Erb's Palsy , the attitude of the limb is _____.
    a. Shoulder add.-Int. rotation-elbow straight
    b. Shoulder add.-Ext. rotation-elbow straight
    c. Shoulder add.-Int. rotation-elbow flexed
    d. None of the above

147. Ape thumb deformity occurs due to the involvement of _____.
    a. Ulna nerve
    b. Median nerve
    c. Radial nerve
    d. Musculocutaneous nerve e

148. The EMG activity of denervation are the following except.
    a. Fibrillation potential
    b. Positive sharp wave
    c. Polyphasic action potential
    d. All of the above

149. Increased polyphasic action potential is a feature of_____.
    a. Dennervation
    b. Polymyositis
    c. Myasthenia gravis
    d. Myopathy

150. Electrodiagnosis of nerve injury should be initiated after —————.
    a. 1 week
    b. 2 week
    c. 4 week
    d. 6 week

151. Exploration after nerve injury is done, if no recovery occurs, after————months.
    a. 2-3
    b. 3-4
    c. 5-6
    d. 12

152. Meralgia parasthetica occurs in———————— nerve.
    a. Sciatic
    b. Superficial peroneal
    c. Lateral femoral cutaneous
    d. Sural

153. What is the minimum time by which the severed axons begins to send out a greater number of sprouts following injury?
    a. 6 hours
    b. One day
    c. 3 weeks
    d. 2 weeks.

154. After median/ulnar nerve repair at wrist the extension of wrist can begin from _____ week.
    a. 3	b. 4
    c. 6	d. 8
155. Secondary nerve repair is done _____ weeks after injury.
    a. 1-3	b. 3-6
    c. 6-12	d. None of the above
156. The wrist should be kept flexed up to _____ weeks after median and ulnar nerve repair at wrist
    a. 2	b. 3
    c. 4	d. 6
157. Nerve conduction velocity for upper limb nerves are ___ _____.
    a. 40-50 m/sec	b. 50-70 m/sec
    c. 70-90 m/sec	d. 90-110 m/sec
158. Nerve conduction velocity for lower limb nerves are___ _____.
    a. 30-45 m/sec	b. 40-55 m/sec
    c. 55-75 m/sec	d. >75 m/sec
159. Normal sensory action potential is _____.
    a. Biphasic	b. Triphasic
    c. Tetraphasic	d. Multiphasic
160. The clinical utility of F wave is to know_____.
    a. Conduction of distal part of nerve
    b. To test the reflex arc
    c. Conduction at proximal part of nerve.
    d. Conduction at neuromuscular junction
161. Latency of F wave for upper limb is _____.
    a. 10-20 msec	b. 12-20 m sec
    c. 20-32 m sec	d. 32-40 m sec
162. Latency of F wave for lower limb is _____.
    a. 10-12 msec	b. 12-25 m sec
    c. 25-42 m sec	d. 42-55 m sec
163. H reflex is electrical equivalent of _____.
    a. Deep tendon reflex
    b. Afferent path of reflex arc
    c. Superficial reflex
    d. Efferent path of reflex

164. Motor end plate of a dennervated muscle persist for _____.
    a. 3 months b. 6 months
    c. 1 year d. 2 years
165. One year after nerve injury the regenerating axon may have ———% reduction in conduction velocity.
    a. 15 b. 25
    c. 35 d. 45
166. In case of Guillain –bare syndrome partial to complete recovery takes usually within _____ months.
    a. Upto 3 b. 3-6
    c. 6-9 d. 9-12
167. All of the factors below are true for the dysthetic pain, which is a type of peripheral neuropathic pain except _____.
    a. Impulse arise from damaged or regenerating nociceptive afferent
    b. Burning type of pain
    c. Paroxysmal shooting/ stabbing present
    d. Pain follow course of a nerve trunk
168. Mechanical allodynia in response to palpation of specific nerve trunk may be due to _____.
    a. Discriminated micro neuroma
    b. Spread of mechano sensitivity along the nerve trunk
    c. All of the above
    d. a and b
169. Physical signs of neuropathic pain include _____.
    a. Antalgic posture
    b. Active and passive movement dysfunction
    c. Adverse response to neural tissue
    d. All of the above
170. The altered production of the bioactive material by vibration due to driving usually of _____ Hz
    a. 5 Hz b. 10 Hz
    c. 15 Hz d. 20 Hz
171. Temporary axonal transport decrease can occur at increase of _____ mm hg pressure which can be easily induced by day to day activity.

a. 10 mm hg b. 30 mm hg
c. 50 mm hg d. 100 mm hg
172. The possible physiological response of neurodynamic test is _____.
    a. Alteration in intra neural blood flow
    b. Axonal transport
    c. Sympathetic activation
    d. All of the above
    e. a and b
173. For uninterrupted blood supply to nerve fibre the pressure gradient should be _____.
    a. Epineural arteriole > capillary fascicle > epineural venule> tunnel
    b. Capillary fascicle > epineural arteriole > epineural venule . tunnel
    c. Tunnel > epineural venule . capillary fascicle > epineural arteriole
    d. None of the above
174. When the tunnel pressure rises to _____ mm Hg venous drainage stops.
    a. > 10 mm hg
    b. 10-20 mm hg
    c. 20- 30 mm hg
    d. 50 mm hg
175. The causes of subclinical nerve injury are_____.
    a. Unphysiological movement
    b. Abnormal body posture
    c. Repetitive muscle contraction
    d. All of the above
    e. b and c
176. The pain characteristics for intra neural conducting tissue involvement _____.
    a. Catches and twinges around vulnerable area
    b. Burning type
    c. Electrical like
    d. Lines of pain
    e. b and c
    f. All of the above

177. Which one among the following is median nerve dominating emphasizing more on shoulder depression and shoulder external rotation ?
    a. ULLT-1   b. ULLT-2
    c. ULTT   d. ULTT-3
    e. None
178. Which one among the following has ulnar nerve bias?
    a. ULTT-1   b. ULTT-2
    c. ULTT-3   d. None
179. During SLR addition of hip medial rotation sensitizes _____.
    a. Tibial division of the sciatic nerve
    b. Peroneal division of sciatic nerve
    c. Sciatic nerve as a whole
    d. Sural nerve
180. The best indicator of disc prolapse is _____.
    a. Bowstring test   b. SLR affected site
    c. Crossed SLR   d. Bilateral SLR
181. Ipsilateral paralysis and dorsal column interruption with contralateral loss of pain and temperature occur in _____.
    a. Central cord syndrome
    b. Anterior cord syndrome
    c. Brown sequard syndrome
    d. Conus medullaris lesion.
182. Patients with SCI lesion T1 and above lose how much respiration function?
    a. 60 % to 80 %   b. 40 % to 50 %
    c. 20 % to 30 %   d. 80 % to 90 %
183. The features of autonomic dysreflexia are_____.
    a. Tachycardia, hypertension, headache
    b. Bradycardia, hypertension, headache
    c. Pallor, tachycardia, headache
    d. All of the above.
184. Which SCI patient among the following will not have an effective cough?
    a. Lesion below T9
    b. Lesion below T6
    c. Lesion Below T1
    d. Conus medullaris lesion.

185. Who is a functional walker among the following SCI?
    a. Lesion Below T6
    b. Lesion below – T9
    c. Lesion below – T10
    d. Lesion below – L1
186. The first superficial reflex to recover following SCI is __.
    a. Bulbocavernous.   b. Anal
    c. Cremasteric   d. Abdominal
187. Crede maneuver is clinically indicated in autonomous bladder, if post-void urine is _____.
    a. Less than 50-100 cc.
    b. Less than 100-120 ccHz.
    c. Less than 120-150 cc
    d. More than 150 cc
188. A young complete SCI patient is having muscle power Hip flexors G4, Add. G4 , Quad. G 4 and other muscles G0; loss of sensation below L3 . Which type of aids will be more appropriate for his ambulation ?
    a. Bil. HKAFO with bil. Axillary crutches
    b. Bil. KAFO with bil. Axillary crutches
    c. Bil. KAFO with bil. Elow crutches
    d. Bil. AFO with bil. elbow crutches
189. Which mode of ambulatory device a SCI patient will use for almost normal speed as well as Oxygen uptake ?
    a. Bil. AFO with bil. elbow crutches
    b. Bil. KAFO with bil. axillary crutches
    c. Bil. HKAFO with bil. Axillary crutches.
    d. Wheel chair.
190. Which is not related to TOURCH?
    a. Tetanjus   b. Rubella
    c. Herpes   d. Cytomegalovirus
191. Diazepam dosage for SCI _____.
    a. Upto 10 mg daily
    b. 6-40 mg daily
    c. 50-100mg daily
    d. None of the above
192. Tenodesis grip is important for_____ level SCI patient.
    a. C5   b. C6
    c. C8   d. T1

193. Which position is used to prepare SCI patient to assume long sitting position?
    a. Prone on hands
    b. Prone on elbows
    c. Supine on hands
    d. Supine on elbows
194. In SCI patient impaired bladder or bowel function or noxious stimulus can produce _____.
    a. Sympathetic over activity
    b. Parasympathetic over activity
    c. Diminished motor activity
    d. None of the above
195. Armrest in wheelchair can support body weight _____.
    a. Above 10%   b. Above 15%
    c. Above 6%   d. Above 5%
196. Most ideal management for bladder is _____.
    a. Indwelling catheter for ever
    b. CIC
    c. External catheter
    d. Crede's maneuver
197. Spinal reflexes are integrated at _____.
    a. 2 months   b. 4 months
    c. 6 months   d. 8 months
198. Moro reflex is _____.
    a. Abduction, extension and internal rotation of arms
    b. Abduction, extension and external rotation of arms
    c. Adduction, internal rotation, extension of arms
    d. Abduction, internal rotation, flexion of arms
199. Fluctuation of muscle tone is found in ——.
    a. Spastic CP   b. Flaccid CP
    c. Athetoid CP   d. None of the above
200. The prenatal cause in cerebral palsy is _____.
    a. Hypertension   b. Diabetes melitus
    c. Torch infection d. Breech presentation
201. Which of the following is most disabling for standing?
    a. Moro   b. Flexor withdrawal
    c. Crossed extension d. Extensor trust

202. Which of the below mentioned primitive reflexes is more disabling for transition from supine to sitting?
    a. ATNR   b. STNR
    c. TLR   d. Moro
203. Which primitive reflex is dangerous for wheelchair bound patients?
    a. ATNR   b. STNR
    c. TLR   d. Crossed extension
204. Brainstem reflexes are integrated in the 1st_____.
    a. 2 months of life   b. 4 months of life
    c. 6 months of life   d. 8 months of life
205. Association reactions are_____ level reflex.
    a. Spinal   b. Mid brain
    c. Brainstem   d. Cortical
206. Righting and equilibrium start developing at the age of__.
    a. 1 year   b. 6 months
    c. 1 ½ years   d. 2 years
207. Righting is_____ level reflex.
    a. Midbrain   b. Cortical
    c. Cerebellar   d. None of the above
208. While putting the child in prone lying position all the position described below are correct except_____.
    a. Shoulder and hips at right angles in weight bearing position.
    b. Knee pointing outward.
    c. Shoulder and arms turned inward
    d. Hands open and palms down
209. Bunny hopping can be discouraged by _____.
    a. Providing prone board with caster
    b. Providing a tricycle
    c. Training bottom shuffle
    d. a and b
    e. a ,b and c
210. Normally child can bridge hips at _____.
    a. 3 months   b. 3-6 months
    c. 5-9 months   d. 7-10 months
211. For children who are excessively extended in supine position, which is the best position to rise them to sitting?

a. Train them to come diagonally from supine
b. Train them to come to sitting straight
c. Train them to come from side lying
d. All of the above

212. The treatment for patients with apraxia is to _____.
    a. Provide tactile, kinesthetic and proprioceptive input
    b. Perform activity in usual environment
    c. Use goal directed activity
    d. Keep command with minimum wordiness
    e. All of the above

213. Chair sitting may be encouraged than floor sitting for all except _____.
    a. Athetoid
    b. With poor sitting balance
    c. With tight hamstring
    d. For young babies

214. Which one among the following is less effective in improving the weight bearing on affected side in hemiplegia?
    a. Moving a small trolly backward and forward with affected leg
    b. Standing , taking the affected leg backward to cross the leg
    c. Stepping backward
    d. Walking with arms held back

215. The most common cause of stroke is _____.
    a. Ischemia
    b. Haemorrhagic
    c. Subarachnoid hemorrhage
    d. Aneurysm

216. In which type of stroke the full extent of insult is apparent from outset?
    a. Haemorrhage   b. Ischaemia
    c. Aneurysm   d. None

217. Anterior cerebral artery lesion will result in _____.
    a. Ipsilateral lower limb sensory loss
    b. Ipsilateral upper limb sensory loss
    c. Contralateral lower limb sensory loss
    d. Both upper limb and lower limb sensory loss

218. Middle cerebral artery lesion will result in
    a. Ipsilateral sensory loss of whole trunk
    b. Contralateral sensory loss of upper limb, lower limb and face
    c. Contralateral sensory loss of upper limb.
    d. None
219. The most prominent symptoms following posterior cerebral artery occlusion is _____.
    a. Auditory   b. Apraxia
    c. Visual   d. Motor
220. Patients with subcortical lesion will have _____.
    a. Loss of sensation of upper limb contralateral
    b. Loss of sensation of upper limb and lower limb contralateral
    c. Loss of sensation upper limb, lower limb and face contralateral
    d. Loss of sensation of upper limb, lower limb, trunk and face
221. Parietal lobe lesion exhibit _____.
    a. Lack of sensory motor integration
    b. Inability to interpret meaningful sensory information
    c. Both a and b.   d. None
222. Which is the critical period of stroke rehabilitation?
    a. Acute stage
    b. Intermediate stage
    c. Discharge and transfer stage
    d. Long term
223. Massed practice in practice time is _____.
    a. Equal to rest   b. More than rest
    c. Less than rest   d. None
224. Blocked practice is _____.
    a. Different tasks done one by one
    b. Consistent practice of single task
    c. Varying tasks one by one
    d. None
225. Crossed hemiplegia occurs when lesion is
    a. Above pontine
    b. At the level of pontine

c. Below pontine
d. None of the above
226. According to Bobath's NDT _____.
    a. Postural control must be restored before limb control
    b. Limb movements should be practiced before development of axial control
    c. Normal movements should be given over abnormal tone
    d. Abnormal synergy can be used to re-educate normal movements
227. Which of the following is inhibitory in NDT?
    a. Passive weight shifting
    b. Active weight shifting
    c. Joint traction –approximation
    d. Tapping
228. To develop upper extremity control by NDT approach priority is given for ___.
    a. Dissociation of scapula from thorax
    b. Shoulder movements should be initiated first
    c. Distal control has to be developed first
    d. None of the above
229. Which of the following is correct regarding motor learning?
    a. Absolute errors are smaller for variable practice than constant practice
    b. Performance is better in blocked practice during acquisition phase, whereas performance is better in random practice during transfer phase.
    c. Distributed practice improves performance is better than massed practice
    d. All of the above
230. Infarction in angular gyrus will lead to _____ apraxia.
    a. Anmesic   b. Global
    c. Conduction   d. Pair word deafness
231. Motor behaviour follows sensory stimulus is the assumption of _____ approach.
    a. Bobath   b. Brunstorm
    c. Rood's   d. PNF

232. Which neurological approach is exclusively applied for stroke patients?
    a. Bobath   b. Brunstorm
    c. Rood's   d. Motor learning
233. In which neurological approach the associated movement can be used to facilitate movement?
    a. Bobath   b. Brunstorm
    c. Motor relearning d. Rood's
234. Normalize tone ,movement, posture is the assumption of _____ approach?
    a. Bobath   b. Brunstorm
    c. Rood's   d. Motor relearning
235. There are _____ stages of recovery according to Brunstorm approach?
    a. 4   b. 5
    c. 6   d. 7
236. Key point control described in _____ approach.
    a. Brunstorm   b. Bobath
    c. Knot and Voss   d. Rood's
237. Interaction of individual, task, environment is described by _____.
    a. Knot and VOSS   b. Bobath
    c. Brunstorm   d. Car and Sephard
238. Glasgow coma scale has _____ points
    a. 12   b. 10
    c. 8   d. 15
239. Severe brain damage scoring in Glasgow coma scale is _____.
    a. < 8   b. < 10
    c. < 5   d. <15
240. Glassgow coma scale has _____ subcales.
    a. 2   b. 3
    c. 4   d. 5
241. In mild head injury Glasgow coma scale score is _____.
    a. 9-12   b. 10-14
    c. 13-15   d. 10-15
242. For severe head injury the duration of coma is _____.
    a. >3 Hours   b. >6 Hours
    c. >12 Hours   d. >24 Hours

243. The cardinal late symptoms of head injury are _____.
    a. Headache, vomiting, visual defect
    b. Headache, giddiness, mental disturbance
    c. Vomiting, mental disturbance, visual defect
    d. None of the above
244. Brain death may be _____.
    a. Irreversible loss of capacity for conciousness
    b. Loss of capacity to breathe
    c. Brainstem death
    d. Death of cortex
245. We sleep when _____.
    a. Cortex relaxes
    b. Influence of reticular formation on cortex fails
    c. Sleep center in hypothalamus slows down
    d. None of the above
246. Sleep apnea can occur due to _____.
    a. Lesion in the brainstem
    b. Upper air way obstruction
    c. obesity
    d. a and b
    e. a, b and c
247. The factor which distinguishes between stroke and epilepsy is _____.
    a. Duration of unconsciousness
    b. Existence of adequate cause for fainting
    c. Epilepsy needs external stimulus to occur
    d. Epilepsy is associated with muscular rigidity
248. Catatonia, the result of lesion in basal pons
    a. The patients lacks the impulse to move although not paralyzed
    b. Patient is paralyzed but able to move to some extent
    c. Patient is paralyzed so does not move
    d. None of the above.
249. In persistent vegetative state _____.
    a. Pons functions spared
    b. Pons function lost
    c. Brain stem function spared
    d. Brain stem function lost

250. Cerebral perfusion pressure CPP is equal to_____.
   a. Mean BP + ICP
   b. Mean BP − ICP
   c. ICP − BP
   d. None
251. Which one of the following has minimal underlying brain injury?
   a. Subdural haematoma
   b. Extra dural haematoma
   c. Intra cerebral haematoma
   d. None
252. Choose the correct answer regarding recovery following brain injury.
   a. Slowly developing lesion causes less functional loss than quickly developed lesion
   b. A single larger lesion cause more functional loss than similar lesion produced over time
   c. Restricted person recovers better than the enriched person
   d. Prognosis of injury to a immature brain is better than matured brain
253. How do drugs help in brain injury?
   a. It replaces neurotransmitters
   b. Resolves edema and improves blood circulation
   c. Prevents effects of toxic substances liberated by the dead cells and blocks the effects of free radicals
   d. All of the above
254. Recovery of function following CNS lesion is due to__.
   a. Resolution edema and restoration of blood circulation
   b. Unmasking of silent zones
   c. Neuronal regeneration
   d. All of the above
255. When is ICP monitoring indicated?
   a. If GCS more than 4 midline shift on scan more than 0.5mm and compression
   b. GCS score less than 4, midline shift more than 0.5 mm in CT scan and compression present
   c. GCS less than no compression or midline shift
   d. None

256. Absence of dystrophic occurs in _____.
    a. Dochene muscular dystrophy
    b. Baker muscular dystrophy
    c. Limb girdle muscular dystrophy
    d. All types of myopathy
257. In myopathy which exercise is appropriate?
    a. Low load less repetition
    b. High load high repetition
    c. Low load high repetition
    d. High load low repetition
258. The physical therapy treatment consideration for early middle stage Parkinsonism includes _____.
    a. Preventive exercise programme
    b. Corrective exercise programme
    c. Compensatory and corrective exercise programme
    d. Dementia monitoring
259. The physiological feedback is _____.
    a. Knowledge of result
    b. Knowledge of performance
    c. Open loop   d. Intrinsic
260. Persistence and severe diplopia can be corrected by _____.
    a. Using special glasses
    b. Eye exercises
    c. Patching one eye
    d. By limiting head and neck movement by a soft collar
261. Training new action following tendon transfer is based on_____ learning.
    a. Classic conditioning
    b. Trail and Error learning
    c. Instrumental learning
    d. Procedural learning
262. Frenkel's exercise should be prescribed for————.
    a. Cerebellar ataxia   b. Vestibular ataxia
    c. Sensory ataxia   d. All of the above
263. Which PNF technique is advocated for parkinsonism?
    a. Hold and relax
    b. Rhythmic stabilization

c. Rhythmic initiation
d. All of the above
264. For patients with generalized weakness which test is useful?
   a. Thyroid function
   b. Parathyroid function
   c. Serum cryoglobulin
   d. Serum complement levels
265. Which test is done for myasthenia gravis?
   a. Spinal fluid anlysis
   b. Tensilon
   c. Prolonged fasting test
   d. None of the above

ANSWER SHEET OF PT IN NEUROLOGICAL CONDITIONS

1. c	2. b	3. a	4. a	5. c
6. a	7. c	8. c	9. d	10. c
11. a	12. b	13. b	14. a	15. c
16. a	17. a	18. d	19. c	20. a
21. b	22. b	23. b	24. d	25. b
26. c	27. b	28. c	29. a	30. a
31. a	32. a	33. a	34. b	35. a
36. b	37. b	38. b	39. a	40. c
41. a	42. d	43. c	44. b	45. a
46. e	47. d	48. d	49. b	50. d
51. c	52. a	53. b	54. e	55. b
56. c	57. a	58. b	59. a	60. c
61. c	62. b	63. a	64. a	65. b
66. b	67. b	68. c	69. b	70. e
71. b	72. c	73. b	74. d	75. b
76. c	77. a	78. b	79. a	80. d
81. a	82. c	83. d	84. c	85. a
86. d	87. b	88. a	89. b	90. b
91. b	92. c	93. c	94. a	95. b
96. e	97. d	98. a	99. d	100. a
101. a	102. c	103. d	104. b	105. b
106. d	107. c	108. c	109. d	110. d
111. b	112. b	113. d	114. a	115. a

116. d	117. b	118. d	119. a	120. b
121. d	122. c	123. b	124. c	125. d
126. c	127. b	128. b	129. a	130. c
131. d	132. d	133. c	134. c	135. b
136. b	137. a	138. a	139. b	140. a
141. b	142. b	143. b	144. a	145. a
146. a	147. b	148. c	149. d	150. c
151. b	152. c	153. a	154. c	155. b
156. b	157. b	158. b	159. b	160. c
161. c	162. d	163. a	164. c	165. b
166. b	167. d	168. d	169. d	170. a
171. b	172. d	173. a	174. c	175. d
176. e	177. b	178. c	179. b	180. c
181. c	182. b	183. b	184. b	185. c
186. b	187. a	188. d	189. d	190. a
191. b	192. b	193. d	194. a	195. a
196. b	197. a	198. b	199. c	200. c
201. b	202. b	203. c	204. c	205. c
206. b	207. a	208. c	209. e	210. b
211. c	212. e	213. d	214. a	215. a
216. b	217. c	218. b	219. c	220. c
221. a	222. c	223. b	224. b	225. b
226. a	227. a	228. a	229. d	230. a
231. c	232. b	233. b	234. a	235. c
236. b	237. d	238. d	239. a	240. b
241. c	242. b	243. b	244. c	245. b
246. e	247. b	248. a	249. c	250. b
251. b	252. a	253. d	254. d	255. b
256. a	257. c	258. b	259. c	260. c
261. a	262. c	263. c	264. a	265. b

Physiotherapy in Cardiopulmonary Conditions

1. At birth the shape of the chest is
   a. Barrel like   b. Circular
   c. Elliptical   d. Triangular
2. Angle of Louis corresponds to
   a. T2 – T3 spine   b. T4 – T5 spine
   c. T6 – T7 spine   d. None of the above
3. Pump handle movement is a feature of
   a. Lower ribs   b. Upper ribs
   c. Mid ribs   d. Diaphragm
4. Maximum diaphragmatic movement is _____ cm
   a. 1 cm   b. 2 cm
   c. 3 cm   d. 4 cm
5. The position of the lung is up to
   a. T8   b. T10
   c. T12   d. T7
6. Approximately the partial pleura extends _____ ribs below the lung
   a. 1   b. 2   c. 3   d. None of the above

7. Central chemoreceptors are stimulated by
   a. Increased $PaCO_2$
   b. Hypoxia
   c. Decreased $PaCO_2$
   d. SaO_2
8. Lower lobe alveoli operates at
   a. Increased transmural pressure
   b. Decreased transmural pressure
   c. Balanced transmural pressure
   d. None of the above
9. Cost of breathing is high when
   a. Diaphragm is used
   b. Inter costals are used
   c. Abdominals are used
   d. Accessories are used
10. V/Q for normal blood gas is
    a. .8
    b. 1
    c. 1.2
    d. 1.1
11. Till 2 years of age
    a. No pump handle movement
    b. No bucket handle movement
    c. No normal diaphragmatic movement
    d. All of the above
12. The gas exchange area is_____ times more in adults than in children
    a. 12 times
    b. 20 times
    c. 25 times
    d. 15 times
13. O_2 consumption rate for neonate is
    a. Half than adults
    b. Same as adults
    c. Twice as adults
    d. Thrice as adults
14. Heart rate for children is
    a. 100 – 110
    b. 80 – 100
    c. 100 – 180
    d. none of the above
15. Which is the pacemaker of the heart?
    a. SA node
    b. AV node
    c. AV bundle
    d. Purkinje fibres
16. Infant BP is
    a. 80/60
    b. 60/40
    c. 100/80
    d. 120/80

17. False high BP reading will occur if ___.
    a. Cuff is too small
    b. Cuff applied loosely
    c. Brachial artery is lower than the heart level
    d. All of the above
18. Normal lung can withstand how much pressure?
    a. 100 cmH$_2$O   b. 120 cmH$_2$O
    c. 150 cm H$_2$O   d. 200 cmH$_2$O
19. Normal central venous pressure should be between
    a. 0 – 5 mmHg   b. 0 – 10 mmHg
    c. 0 – 15 mmHg   d. 0 – 20 mmHg
20. Normally total cholesterol level is _____.
    a. < 200 mg/dl   b. < 250 mg/dl
    c. < 300 mg/dl   d. < 400 mg/dl
21. Normal cholesterol to HDL ratio is___.
    a. 1-2   b. 2-3
    c. 3-5   d. 5-7
22. Percussion and vibration should be discontinued when PaO$_2$ reaches
    a. 50   b. 55
    c. 65   d. 80
23. Usually suction pressure for adults is
    a. 80 mmHg   b. 100 mmHg
    c. 120 mmHg   d. 70 mmHg
24. Suction times should be less than
    a. 5 seconds   b. 20 seconds
    c. 15 seconds   d. 30 seconds
25. Which is not a complication of suction?
    a. Vagal stimulation   b. Hypotension
    c. Atelectasis   d. Cough
26. Which is not a complication of hyperinflation?
    a. Pneumothorax
    b. Bronchospasm
    c. Increased cardiac output
    d. Decreased cardiac output
27. Pulmonary artery hypertension is when mean PA pressure is
    a. > 10 mmHg   b. > 20 mmHg
    c. > 30 mmHg   d. > 40 mmHg

28. Which is not a risk factor for pulmonary artery hypertension?
    a. Multiple blood transfusion
    b. Chest trauma
    c. Near drowning
    d. Aspiration of gastric content
29. Patients with diffusion problems will have
    a. Normal $PaCO_2$
    b. Hypoxaemia and normal $PaCO_2$
    c. Hypoxaemia and hypercapnia
    d. Normal PaO_2 with hypercapnia
30. In which of the following O_2 therapy will not help
    a. Dead space
    b. Shunt
    c. Respiratory failure
    d. None of the above
31. Shifting of mediastinum to right may occur in
    a. Right collapse
    b. Left collapse
    c. Right pleurisy
    d. None of the above
32. Early inspiratory crackles occur with
    a. Less of compliant airways
    b. More compliant airways
    c. Stiff lung
    d. Obstructed airway
33. Which of the following techniques does not require radiation?
    a. Computerized tomography
    b. Conventional radiography
    c. Magnetic resonance imaging
    d. None of the above
34. Which diagnostic technique is better for differentiation of soft tissue?
    a. X-rays
    b. Ultrasonography
    c. CT scan
    d. MRI

35. The duration at QRS complex is
    a. .12 to .2 sec   b. .08 to .1 sec
    c. .1 to .15 sec   d. .02 to .04 sec
36. The normal running speed of ECG is
    a. 30 mm/sec   b. 20 mm/sec
    c. 25 mm/sec   d. 40mm/sec
37. Which chest lead assess right ventricle
    a. V1,V2   b. V2, V3
    c. V3, V4   d. V5, V6
38. Among the below ECG abnormality which is most dangerous
    a. Atrial fibrillation
    b. Ventricular tachycardia
    c. AV block
    d. Supra ventricular tachycardia
39. Drop of QRS complex is found in
    a. 1st degree heart block
    b. 2nd degree heart block
    c. 3rd degree heart block
    d. both a and b
40. Which is a definitive feature of transmural infarction?
    a. S-T segment elevation
    b. ST segment depression
    c. Abnormal Q
    d. Reduction in R wave
41. Prolonged P-R interval is seen in which type of A-V block
    a. Mobitz-1   b. Mobitz-2
    c. First degree   d. Third degree
42. Duration of QRS complex is____ ms.
    a. 0.04-0.11   b. 0.12-0.20
    c. 0.21 – 0.30   d. None of the above
43. In right ventricular hypertrophy the R wave is largest in which lead
    a. V1   b. V2
    c. V3   d. V4
44. Which ventricular rhythm is known as dying heart?
    a. Ventricular fibrillation
    b. Ventricular tachycardia

c. Idioventricular rythm
   d. None of the above
45. Which is gold standard for diagnosis of myocardial infarction?
   a. ECG b. ECHO
   c. Lipid profile d. Cardiac catheterization
46. Which is not an inotropic drug?
   a. Digoxin b. Dobutamin
   c. Enoximon d. Furosemide
47. Which is a long acting B2 stimulant?
   a. Salbutamol b. Salmetrol
   c. Fenoterol d. Ipratropium bromide
48. Pulmonary artery wedge pressure reflexes
   a. Right atrial pressure
   b. Right ventricular pressure
   c. Left atrial pressure
   d. Left ventricular pressure
49. The patient can be assumed to be hypoxemic in room air if PaO_2 is
   a. $< FIO_2 \times 5$ b. $> FIO_2 \times 5$
   c. $< FIO_2 \times 2$ d. $< FIO_2 \times 3$
50. Patient who is chronically ill with cardiopulmonary disease PaO_2 should not fall below
   a. 40mmHg b. 50mmHg
   c. 60mmHg d. 80mmHg
51. _____ is better compensated with metabolic buffers
   a. Respiratory alkalosis
   b. Respiratory acidosis
   c. Both respiratory acidosis and alkalosis
   d. Non of the above
52. When there is a significant base deficit the appropriate terminology is
   a. Acidosis b. Academia
   c. Alkalemia d. Alkalosis
53. If $PaCO_2 > 50mmHg$ and PH is 7.3 to 7.4 then patient is suffering from which of the following condition
   a. Acute ventilatory failure
   b. Chronic ventilatory failure

c. Partially compensated metabolic alkalosis
d. Compensated metabolic alkalosis

54. Which is better predictor of oxygen saturation?
    a. Pulse oxymetry   b. CO oxymeter
    c. Both a and b   d. None of them

55. If patients minute volume is half of the normal value approximate $PaCO_2$ is
    a. 40 mmHg   b. 50mmHg
    c. 60 mmHg   d. 70 mmHg

56. Which of the following will not shift the oxyhaemoglobin dissociation curve to right?
    a. Acute acidosis
    b. Acute alkalosis
    c. High carbondioxide
    d. Increased temperature

57. When using 70 % helium and 30 % O_2 and observed flow is 10L/min. then actual flow is
    a. 10 X1.1 = 11L/min
    b. 10 x 1.5 = 15L/min
    c. 10 X 1.6 = 16L/min
    d. 10 X 1.8 = 18L/min

58. While using venture mask the total flow through the mask should be
    a. 2 – 3 times minute volume
    b. 3 – 4 times minute volume
    c. 4 – 6 times minute volume
    d. 8 – 10 times minute volume

59. Simple oxygen mask with a flow of 5 to 10L/min provide
    a. 20 % to 30 % FiO_2 b. 30 – 50 %
    c. 35 % to 60%   d. 60 % to 80%

60. The recommended frequency of performing incentive spirometry is
    a. 4 times/day
    b. 5 times/hour while awake
    c. 10 times/day
    d. 10 times/hour while awake

61. For humidification which is the most important concept
    a. Absolute humidity
    b. Vapor pressure
    c. Body humidity
    d. Relative humidity
62. Humidity should be added to the flow when it is
    a. > 4 L/min   b. > 2 L/min
    c. > 10 L/min   d. > 6 L/min
63. Diaphragm functioning is tested clinically by
    a. Maximum breathing capacity
    b. Inspiratory strength measurement
    c. Measuring VC in supine and sitting
    d. Both a and b
64. When patient breathe at low lung volume
    a. Base is better ventilated than apex
    b. Apex is better ventilated than base
    c. Apex and base equally ventilated
    d. V/Q = 1
65. For hypoxaemic patient which position will you prefer
    a. Supine   b. Side lying
    c. Prone   d. Prone abdomen free
66. Forced expiratory technique is
    a. Mid lung volume huff – diaphragmatic breathing – cough
    b. High lung volume huff – diaphragmatic breathing – cough
    c. Low – mid lung volume huff – diaphragmatic breathing – cough
    d. None of the above
67. A sequence of breathing at volumes and flow rate
    a. FET   b. ACBT
    c. Autogenic drainage   d. Both a and b
68. Which is not a self drainage procedure
    a. FET   b. ACBT
    c. Autogenic drainage   d. Prone on elbow
69. Flutter is a
    a. High frequency PEP device
    b. Chest compressor
    c. Vibrator
    d. None of the above

70. Pressure at umbilicus by heel of the palm is
    a. Costophrenic assist
    b. Helmich type assist
    c. Anterior chest compression assist
    d. None of the above
71. Which all are the movement strategies associated with inspiration
    a. Shoulder flexion, abduction, external rotation
    b. Shoulder flexion, trunk extension up to eye gaze
    c. Shoulder flexion, abduction, external rotation, trunk extension, eye gaze
    d. Trunk extension, shoulder flexion, abduction, external rotation
72. Out of bed activities are contraindicated when patient is connected to
    a. Oxygen cylinder
    b. Bed side monitor
    c. Intra aortic balloon pump
    d. All of the above three
73. $PaCO_2$ is
    a. Directly proportional to ventilation
    b. Inversely proportional to ventilation
    c. Directly proportional to blood pH
    d. Inversely proportional to blood pH
74. If $PaCO_2$ is within (30-50) mmHg and pH>7.5 then there is
    a. Respiratory acidosis
    b. Metabolic alkalosis
    c. Respiratory alkalosis
    d. Acceptable ventilatory and metabolic status
75. The relationship of pH with $PaCO_2$ is
    a. For every 20mmHg rise in $PaCO_2$ decrease the pH by 0.10
    b. For every 20mmHg rise in $PaCO_2$ increase the pH by 0.10
    c. For every 10mmHg rise in $PaCO_2$ decrease the pH by 0.10
    d. For every 20mmHg fall in $PaCO_2$ increase the pH by 0.10

76. Patients with high functional capacity but low reserve need
    a. Shorter training course
    b. Longer training course
    c. Progressive training course
    d. None of the above
77. Which of the following will not help to produce cough?
    a. Application of ice below axilla
    b. Extra thoracic tracheal pressure
    c. Manual ventilation
    d. Change of position
78. Equal pressure point in low lung volume remains at
    a. Trachea   b. Lobar bronchi
    c. Alveoli   d. Segmental bronchi
79. At what phase of cough the intra thoracic pressure rises to the maximum during
    a. Inspiratory phase
    b. Glottic closure
    c. Contraction of expiratory muscles
    d. Expiratory phase
80. The frequency of manual vibration is
    a. 5 – 12 Hz   b. 12 – 20 Hz
    c. 20 – 25 Hz   d. None of the above
81. Vibrations should be less vigorous for patients with
    a. Lung abscess   b. Chronic bronchitis
    c. # Thoracic spine   d. Asthma
82. Which is not true for percussion?
    a. It is done with fingers and thumb adducted
    b. The sound of percussion should be hollow sound
    c. The rate of percussion between 100-475 times per minute.
    d. The dominant hand pressure is more than non dominant hand
83. For low pressure PEP therapy the resistance is adjusted till the PEP level is
    a. 5-10 cm H_2O
    b. 10-20 cm H_2O
    c. Forced vital capacity pressure
    d. None of the above

84. An indicator of effective cough is when FEV_1 is at least
    a. 40% of VC
    b. 60% of VC
    c. 80% of VC
    d. 50% of VC
85. For every cigarette an individual smoke the cilia are paralyzed for
    a. 5 minutes
    b. 10 minutes
    c. 20 minutes
    d. 30 minutes
86. Which one among the following is not an self assisted technique for cough?
    a. Prone on elbows head flexion
    b. Hands knee rocking
    c. Counter rotation
    d. Short sitting
87. The muscular work of breathing is _____ % of total body oxygen consumption
    a. 5%
    b. 10%
    c. 15%
    d. 20%
88. Patients with secondary pulmonary dysfunction need to
    a. Relax their accessory muscle and use diaphragm more
    b. Balance the use of diaphragm and accessory muscle
    c. Reduce the work of breathing
    d. None of the above
89. Re-patterning technique is used for
    a. COPD cases
    b. Patients with short of breath
    c. Patients with high respiratory rate
90. Patients with accumulation of secretion 4 gm of carbohydrate produces _____ Kcal
    a. 6.2 Kcal
    b. 4.2 K cal
    c. 3.2 K cal
    d. 9.2 K cal
91. For a mixed diet, for each litre of oxygen consumed how much energy is produced
    a. 8 K cal
    b. 6 K cal
    c. 5 K cal
    d. 4 K cal
92. Resting oxygen consumption expenditure for a 60 Kg man is _____
    a. 2 litres
    b. 0.2 litres
    c. 0.5 litres
    d. 5 litres

93. 1 litre of oxygen expended is equivalent to how much calories
    a. 10 K cal
    b. 10 cal
    c. 5 cal
    d. 5 K cal
94. In monark cycle ergometre for each revolution how much distance is traveled
    a. 5 m
    b. 6 m
    c. 3 m
    d. 2 m
95. Kreb cycle takes place in
    a. Cytoplasm
    b. Mitochondria
    c. Outside cell
    d. Ribosome
96. In a interval training the metabolic response of 2nd exercise is similar to the first if the interval is
    a. .5 – 1 min
    b. 1 – 2 min
    c. Within 2 minutes
    d. Can never be same
97. For graded exercise test the increment of exercise should be of
    a. 1 MET
    b. 2 MET
    c. 0.5 MET
    d. 2.5 MET
98. Ideal test time of graded exercise test should be
    a. Within 10 minutes
    b. 5 – 15 minutes
    c. 12 – 16 minutes
    d. 10 – 20 minutes
99. For exercise induced bronchospasm the exercise test should be done in
    a. 1 stage
    b. 2 stages
    c. 3 stages
    d. 4 stages
100. Anaerobic threshold corresponds to _____ % of maximum heart rate
    a. 50 %
    b. 60 %
    c. 75 %
    d. 80 %
101. According to karvonen method training heart rate is _____ % of heart rate reserve
    a. 40 % to 60 %
    b. 40 % to 85 %
    c. 50 % to 75 %
    d. None of the above
102. In 20 point scale of rate of perceived exertion 12 – 13 score corresponds to
    a. 50 % of HRR
    b. 60 % of HRR
    c. 85 % of HRR
    d. 30 % of HRR

103. In 10 point scale of RPE 60 % of HRR corresponds to
    a. 4
    b. 6
    c. 5
    d. 3
104. Average duration of cardiac rehabilitation as outpatient is
    a. 8 weeks
    b. 12 weeks
    c. 16 weeks
    d. 20 weeks
105. The frequency of exercise training is _____ when MET is 3 – 5
    a. 3 – 5 times/weeks
    b. 2 – 3 times/weeks
    c. 4 – 6 times/weeks
    d. Every day
106. During aerobic training how long does it take for conditioning
    a. 4 – 6 weeks
    b. 2 – 4 weeks
    c. 6 – 10 weeks
    d. 8 – 12 weeks
107. The improvement in aerobic training continues in an average for
    a. 2 – 3 months
    b. 3 – 4 months
    c. 4 – 5 months
    d. 10 months
108. PcO_2 to PaO_2 is
    a. Ventilation dependent
    b. Diffusion dependent
    c. Ventilation – perfusion dependent
    d. Perfusion dependent
109. Dead space ventilation in ml is
    a. 2 X body weight in kg
    b. 1.5 X body weight in kg
    c. 3 X body weight in kg
    d. Same as body weight in kg
110. During exercise the dead space
    a. Increases
    b. Decreases
    c. Remains same as resting
111. During moderate to high exercise how does ventilation increase
    a. By increasing breathing frequency
    b. By increasing tidal volume
    c. By increasing tidal volume and breathing frequency
    d. By decreasing dead space

112. When mitral stenosis patient exercise the muscles can extract upto what % of CO
    a. 40 %   b. 30 %
    c. 50 %   d. 60 %
113. After loud of heart is controlled by
    a. Aorta   b. Large arteries
    c. Medium arteries d. Arterioles
114. Free fatty acid utilization is better when exercising at
    a. < 50 % of VO_2 max
    b. < 40 % of VO_2 max
    c. < 75 % of VO_2 max
    d. < 60 % of VO_2 max
115. Walking 2 mph requires _____ MET
    a. 1   b. 2
    c. 3   d. 4
116. During self care evaluation in phase I of cardiac rehabilitation heart rate should not exceed
    a. 60/min   b. 100/min
    c. 150/min   d. 75/min
117. At the end of phase II of cardiac rehabilitation which exercise test is done
    a. Bruce protocol
    b. Low level exercise test
    c. Symptom limited end point exercise
    d. Balke
118. The job taken by cardiac patient should be within how much extra O_2 uptake on the resting O_2 uptake
    a. 10 % of reserve
    b. 10 – 20 % of reserve
    c. 25 % to 30 % of reserve
    d. > 50 % of reserve
119. To get central effect the training heart rate should resting HR added with how much % reserve
    a. 60 %   b. 75 %
    c. 50 %   d. 90 %
120. In case of SCI when the diaphragm is innervated but the intercostals and abdominals are paralyzed the aim of breathing exercise is to
    a. Encourage use of diaphragm

b. Diaphragm should be used to its maximum
c. Diaphragm action is kept in check
121. To inhibit diaphragm which position is safer
    a. Prone on elbows
    b. Semi sitting
    c. Semi sitting with anterior pelvic tilt
    d. None of the above
122. What is the best position of ventilation for asymmetrical involvement of chest?
    a. Lying on uninvolved side
    b. Lying on uninvolved side with arms below 90 degrees of shoulder flexion
    c. Lying on involved side
    d. Lying on involved side with arms below 90 degrees of shoulder flexion
123. The effective prescription for chronic arterial occlusion are the following except
    a. Warm outer foot wear in winter
    b. Use of rocker sole shoe
    c. Active graded exercise
    d. Passive limb positioning exercise
124. Sclerotherapy is used for
    a. Acute venous insufficiency
    b. Chronic venous insufficiency
    c. Lymphatic disease
    d. None of the above
125. To do secretion clearance programme at home for an adult patient which one among the following should be preferred?
    a. Postural drainage
    b. Forced expiratory technique
    c. Active cycle of breathing technique
    d. Autogenic drainage
126. Patient with strong diaphragm but no muscular support from intercostals and abdominal muscles may develop
    a. Flattened anterior chest wall
    b. Pectus excavatum
    c. Anterolateral flaring of the lower rib cage
    d. Thoracic kyphosis

127. The physiology of force expiratory technique is based on
    a. Decreased followed by increased airway pressure
    b. Equal pressure point on the airway
    c. Change of volume of ventilation leads to increased pressure in the airway
    d. None of the above
128. When high flow oxygen delivery system is preferred?
    a. When the total inspiratory requirement is not required to be met
    b. When FiO_2 50% can keep SaO_2 at the safe level
    c. Excessive work of breathing
    d. Excessive myocardial work
129. Risk of atelectasis is more when
    a. CV> FRC   b. FRC> CV
    c. CV = FRC   d. CV = TV
130. PEEP of _____ cm H_2O will cause pneumothorax
    a. 10-20 cm H_2O b. 20-30 cmH_2O
    c. 20 – 40 cm H_2O d. 40 – 60 cm H_2O
131. For adults CPAP can be given upto
    a. 2 cm$H_2$0   b. 5 cmH_2O
    c. 8 cmH_2O d. 10 cmH_2O
132. Normal PEEP is
    a. 5 – 10 cm of H_2O b. 5 cm H_2O
    c. 15 – 20 cm H_2O d. 20 – 25 cm H_2O
133. In acute respiratory failure how much tidal volume will decrease the shunting
    a. 8 ml/kg body weight
    b. 10 ml/kg body weight
    c. 5 ml/kg body weight
    d. 15 ml/kg body weight
134. At what pressure in PEEP cardiac output will start to decrease?
    a. 5 cm H_2O b. 10 cm H_2O
    c. 15 cm H_2O d. 20 cm H_2O
135. Which is a sign of oxygen toxicity?
    a. Dyspnoea   b. Substernal pain
    c. Productive cough   d. None of the above

136. The early postoperative complications of heart transplantation are
    a. Rejection
    b. Infection
    c. Right ventricular failure
    d. a and b
    e. a, b, and c
137. The respiratory rate, cycle and TV vary considerably in
    a. Kussamaul's respiration
    b. Biot's respiration
    c. Cheyne – stokes respiration
    d. None of the above
138. Pulsus paradoxus can occur due to the following conditions except
    a. Asthma
    b. Pericardial effusion
    c. Upper airway obstruction
    d. Pneumonia
139. When BP fluctuates _____ mmHg during respiratory cycle of is known as pulsus paradoxus
    a. 8 mmHg   b. 10 mmHg
    c. 15 mmHg   d. 5 mmHg
140. Pulsus alternans with normal heart rate indicates____.
    a. Preventricular contraction
    b. Left ventricular failure
    c. Cardiogenic shock
    d. Cardiomyopathy
141. Which is not a feature of decreased oxygenation?
    a. Bradypnea   b. Tachypnoea
    c. Tachycardia   d. Clubbing
142. A – a gradient of oxygen changes with the following
    a. Position   b. Age
    c. FiO_2 d. All of the above
143. In case of equivocal CVP if 100ml of blood is transfused and BP does not raise then it is
    a. Hypovolemia   b. Hypervolemia
    c. Heart failure   d. Fluid imbalance

144. Usually how much is the 1st hour blood loss after cardiac surgery
    a. 1ml/kg/hr   b. 2ml/kg/hr
    c. 2 – 3ml/kg/hr   d. 4 – 5ml/kg/hr
145. Usually which patients are extubated from the operation theatre except
    a. COA   b. PDA
    c. Closed heart surgery d. VSD
146. Pressure support ventilator triggers with as low as ____ cm of H_2O
    a. 2   b. 5
    c. 10   d. 15
147. Ventilators brings down haemodynamics by around
    a. 10 %   b. 20 %
    c. 30 %   d. 50 %
148. In ventilation the set respiratory rate in adults is usually _____ min
    a. 10 – 12   b. 12 – 18
    c. 20 – 22   d. None of the above
149. When $PaCO_2$ is increased the following should be done except
    a. Increase mechanical deadspace
    b. Decrease mechanical dead space
    c. Increase tidal volume
    d. Increase respiratory rate
150. When the patient can be kept in SIMV
    a. If 50 % FiO_2 kept for ½ an hour ABG – normal
    b. 70 % FiO_2 – for 1 hr – ABG normal
    c. 70 % FiO_2 for ½ an hour ABG – Normal
    d. None of the above
151. Which one among the following is a correct procedure for the process of extubation
    a. Chest PT, Secretion, clean oral cavity remove giggle while doing suction tube
    b. Remove giggle, chest PT, suction which doing suction remove the tube
    c. Chest PT, remove giggle suction and while suctioning takeout the tube
    d. None of the above

152. The 2nd phase of CPR is
    a. Reoxygenate CNS
    b. ABC technique
    c. To restart circulation and definitive treatment
    d. To gauge recovery
153. Which is a disease of acinus?
    a. Bronchitis   b. Asthma
    c. Emphysema   d. Pneumonia
154. A reduction of _____ % from normal lung volumes and capacities may be considered as abnormal
    a. > 10 %   b. > 15 %
    c. > 25 %   d. > 30 %
155. Vital capacity is _____ % of TLC
    a. 60%   b. 70 %
    c. 80 %   d. 90 %
156. Which is not true for peak flow measurement?
    a. It increases with height
    b. It decreases with age
    c. Measured at the end of FVC
    d. Measured at beginning of FVC
157. The uniformity of ventilation is tested by
    a. Measuring carbon monoxide transfer factor
    b. Measuring nitrogen concentration after inspiration of 100% O_2
    c. Measuring O_2 after 100% O_2 inspiration
    d. Measuring transpulmonary pressure
158. FEV1, FVC ratio may increase in
    a. Airway disease
    b. Obstructive airway disease
    c. Restrictive airway disease
    d. Interstitial airway diseases
159. Which finding is typical of lung fibrosis?
    a. TLC, reduced
    b. RV, TLC reduced
    c. RV/TLC ratio reduced
    d. RCO reduced
160. Which is not a combination of obstructive and restrictive defect?
    a. Pulmonary edema

b. Sarcoidosis
   c. Patients on long term steroids for COPD
   d. Bronchiectasis
161. FEV1 less than _____ % is a risk for surgery
   a. 30 %   b. 50 %
   c. 25 %   d. None of the above
162. The cause of bronchial breath sound is
   a. Narrowing of airway
   b. Attenuation of breath sound
   c. Decreased ventilation
   d. None of the above
163. Stony dullness of on percussion is found in
   a. Atelectasis   b. Consolidation
   c. Pleural effusion d. Bronchial asthma
164. At 45^0 recumbent position normal JVP should be
   a. 3 – 4cm   b. 5 – 6cm
   c. 7 – 8cm   d. 10 cm
165. Pneumonia can be termed.
   a. COPD
   b. RestrictiveLungDisease
   c. Interstitial lung disease
   d. Infective lung disease
166. Bullae are seen in
   a. Asthma
   b. Pulmonary embolism
   c. Cor pulmonale
   d. Emphysema
167. Irreversible distortion of the air way is seen in
   a. Bronchitis   b. Pneumonia
   c. Bronchiactasis   d. Emphysema.
168. Croup is inflammation of
   a. Pharynx and larynx   b. Glottis
   c. Larynx and trachea   d. Trachea
169. The value of resting metabolic rate (O_2 uptake) which is called 1 MET is
   a. 3.5 ml/kg/min   b. 3.7 ml/kg/min
   c. 4.5 ml/kg/min   d. 4.7 ml/kg/min
170. The recommended BMI range is from
   a. 14.5 to 17.5 kg/m^2 b. 18.5 to 24.9 kg/m^2
   c. 25.00 to 29.9kg/m^2 d. 30.00 to 35 kg/m^2

171. CRF (cardiorespiratory fitness) value is expressed in the following way
    a. Litres of O_2 used by the body per minute (L/min)
    b. Milli litres of oxygen used per kilogram of body weight per minute.(ml/kg/min)
    c. Multiples of resting metabolic rate (MET).
    d. All of the above.
172. Goose neck deformity is found in
    a. ASD   b. VSD
    c. AP window   d. PDA
173. In low cardiac output syndrome _____
    a. BP is high   b. BP is low
    c. Urinary output is high
    d. Peripheral and core temperature are equal.
174. Cardic pain does not reffered ____.
    a. Above the ear
    b. Below the umbilicus
    c. Above the ear and below the umbilicus
    d. To the opposite shoulder
175. Commonest embolus originates from
    a. DVT   b. Varicose veins
    c. Fat   d. Air
176. Thrombophlebitis _____
    a. Develops silently
    b. Develops in superficial vessels
    c. Develops in deep vessles
    d. Usually give rise to embolism
177. Drainage bottle must be placed
    a. Lower than the patient
    b. Higher than thepatient
    c. Same level
    d. None of the above
178. The swing of fluid level in the glass and piece of drainage bottle is absent when
    a. Lung is fully expanded
    b. Tube is blocked
    c. All of the above
    d. None of the above.

179. The drainage tube should be kept _____ cm under water
    a. 5cm b. 4cm
    c. 2.5cm d. 1.5cm
180. In which surgery chest tube is not given
    a. Lobectomy b. Segmentectomy
    c. Pneumonectomy d. Thoracoplasty
181. Tension sutures are used in
    a. Thoracotomy b. Thoracolasty
    c. Pneumonectomy d. Hernia repair
182. Removal of the whole lung is called
    a. Thoarcotomy b. Thoracoplasty
    c. Skeve Resection d. Pneumonectomy
183. Suitable body position for a post-operative hypoxic patient is
    a. 30 degrees head down
    b. Supine with head and body aligned in neutral.
    c. 30 degrees inclined upward
    d. 60 degrees inclined upward.
184. pH is 7.30, $PaCO_2$ 60mm and Bicarbonate is within normal limit. The condition is _____
    a. Acute respiratory alkalosis
    b. Acute respiratory acidosis
    c. Compensatory respiratory acidosis
    d. Metabolic acidosis
185. Extended sternotomy is done for _____
    a. CABG
    b. Bypass for descending aorta
    c. CMV
    d. ASD
186. Which is desirable for a postoperative case?
    a. CV>FRC b. FRC>CV
    c. CV>TV d. None of the above
187. Bronchopulmonary fistula is a complication following _____
    a. Thoracotomy b. Lobectomy
    c. Thoracoplasty d. Pneumonectomy

188. Which is the most painful thoracic incision?
    a. Sternotomy
    b. Posterolateral thoracotomy
    c. Thoracoabdominal
    d. Anterolateral thoracotomy
189. Immediately following pneumonectomy patient should be positioned in _____
    a. Side lying on operated side
    b. Side lying on sound side
    c. Supine lying
    d. Half lying
190. Complications of pneumonectomy include _____
    a. Mediastinal shift
    b. Bronchopulmonary fistula
    c. Injury to phrenic nerve and recurrent laryngeal nerve
    d. All of the above.
191. In VSD surgery is indicated when PAH is
    a. > 30 %   b. > 20 %
    c. > 50 %   d. > 80 %
192. Which is not an effect of cardio pulmonary bypass?
    a. Interstitial edema
    b. Pleural effusion
    c. Diaphragmatic dysfunction
    d. Pneumothorax
193. Corrective surgery for large VSD should be done within
    a. 5 years   b. 2 years
    c. Infancy   d. 10 years
194. Which one of the congenital heart disease will not show (lt) to (rt) shunt?
    a. VSD   b. VSD with PS
    c. ASD   d. PDA
195. Which cardiac condition can be treated as a closed procedure?
    a. ASD   b. VSD
    c. PDA   d. AP window
196. Which surgery is done for transposition of great vessels?
    a. PA banding   b. Atrial switch
    c. Glenn   d. Fontan

162 Physiotherapy Secrets

197. Which defect is not included in Tetralogy of Fallot?
   a. ASD
   b. VSD
   c. PS
   d. Ventricular hypertrophy
198. BT shunt is between
   a. Descending aorta and left pulmonary artery
   b. Ascending aorta and right pulmonary artery
   c. Subclavian artery with pulmonary artery
   d. Central aorta and pulmonary artery.
199. A flap in the visceral pleura is the cause of
   a. Closed pneumothorax
   b. Open pneumothorax
   c. Tension pneumothorax
   d. None
200. Blunt cardiac injury can occur in
   a. Steering wheel injury
   b. Lap belt injury
   c. Both a and b
   d. None

ANSWER SHEET OF PT IN CARDIO-PULMONARY CONDITIONS

1. b	2. b	3. b	4. c	5. b
6. b	7. a	8. a	9. d	10. b
11. b	12. c	13. c	14. a	15. a
16. b	17. d	18. b	19. b	20. a
21. c	22. b	23. c	24. c	25. d
26. c	27. b	28. b	29. b	30. b
31. a	32. b	33. c	34. d	35. b
36. c	37. a	38. b	39. b	40. c
41. c	42. a	43. a	44. c	45. d
46. d	47. b	48. c	49. a	50. b
51. b	52. a	53. b	54. b	55. b
56. b	57. c	58. c	59. c	60. d
61. d	62. a	63. c	64. b	65. d
66. c	67. c	68. b	69. a	70. b
71. c	72. c	73. b	74. b	75. a
76. b	77. a	78. c	79. c	80. b
81. d	82. d	83. b	84. b	85. c
86. c	87. a	88. b	89. c	90. b

91. c	92. b	93. d	94. b	95. b
96. a	97. a	98. c	99. b	100. c
101. b	102. b	103. a	104. b	105. a
106. a	107. c	108. c	109. a	110. b
111. a	112. c	113. d	114. a	115. b
116. b	117. c	118. c	119. d	120. c
121. b	122. d	123. d	124. b	125. d
126. b	127. b	128. b	129. a	130. c
131. c	132. b	133. d	134. b	135. b
136. e	137. b	138. d	139. b	140. b
141. a	142. d	143. c	144. c	145. d
146. b	147. c	148. b	149. a	150. a
151. a	152. c	153. c	154. b	155. c
156. d	157. b	158. c	159. c	160. d
161. b	162. d	163. c	164. a	165. d
166. d	167. d	168. c	169. a	170. b
171. d	172. a	173. b	174. c	175. a
176. b	177. a	178. c	179. c	180. c
181. d	182. d	183. d	184. b	185. b
186. b	187. d	188. b	189. a	190. a
191. c	192. d	193. b	194. b	195. c
196. b	197. a	198. c	199. c	200. c

Biomechanics

1. Centre of gravity of adult human in the anatomical position is slightly _____.
   a. Anterior to S1 vertebra
   b. Posterior to S1 vertebra
   c. Anterior to S2 vertebra
   d. Posterior to S2 vertebra
2. The centre of gravity of adult human is at about____% of person's height.
   a. 50 %   b. 55 %
   c. 45 %   d. 60 %
3. On unilateral stance the safety zone is limited in _____.
   a. Anteroposterior sway
   b. Side to side sway
   c. Rotatory sway
   d. Both a and b
4. Location of centre of mass of body segment is at _____ % from proximal end.
   a. 40%   b. 50 %
   c. 45 %   d. 55 %
5. Which is not a saddle joint?
   a. Carpometacarpal of thumb
   b. Ankle
   c. Sternocalvicular
   d. Acromioclavicular

6. Normal carrying angle is _____.
   a. 0 - 20
   b. 0 – 30
   c. 0 – 10
   d. 0 – 40
7. The concave – convex rule depicts if the bone with convex joint surface moves on the bone with concavity, the convex joint surface.
   a. Moves in the opposite direction to bone segment
   b. Moves in the same direction to bone segment
   c. Half way in opposite direction and another half way in same direction to bone segment
   d. None
8. Minimal muscle force is required when the joints is on_____.
   a. Closed pack position
   b. Loose pack position
   c. In between close and loose pack position
   d. In extension
9. Newton's 1st law of motion is applicable to which phase of gait cycle?
   a. Stance phase
   b. Swing phase
   c. Mid stance
   d. Push off
10. When two forces applied from one point as the angle between the forces decrease the resultant force_____.
    a. Decrease
    b. Increase
    c. Remains same
    d. Becomes twice
11. The weight on the trunk balanced by the erector spinae muscle in standing is application of which lever system are less.
    a. 1st class
    b. 2nd class
    c. 3rd class
    d. 2nd and 3rd class
12. Which class is lever of power?
    a. 1st
    b. 2nd
    c. 3rd
    d. 2nd and 3rd
13. Joint reaction force is _____.
    a. Compressive force in a joint
    b. Compressive force and muscle compressive force
    c. Compressive force and muscle rotatory force
    d. Compressive force of muscle and other soft tissues

14. Weight of HAT is about _____ % of bodyweight
    a. 40 %   b. 50 %
    c. 60 %   d. 70 %
15. The centre of gravity of HAT is at
    a. T10   b. T11
    c. L1   d. T9
16. The damaging distracting force is found in
    a. Codman's pendulum exercise
    b. Weight attached to foot in osteo arthritis knee
    c. Weight attached to foot in ligament injury
    d. Weight attached for strengthening in ankylosing hip
17. Which is not a anatomical pulley?
    a. FDP contraction
    b. Quadriceps contraction
    c. Hamstring contraction
    d. Peroneal contraction
18. The lever arm of gastrosoleus muscle force at ankle joint is about _____.
    a. 2"   b. 1"
    c. 3"   d. 1.5"
19. Biceps brachii as an elbow flexor is most effective at _____ elbow flexion range.
    a. 45   b. 60
    c. 90   d. 120
20. Which exercises are harmful for RA joint?
    a. Passive stretching   b. Passive mobilization
    c. Active stretching   d. Active mobilization
21. When the muscle is relaxed the length of each sarcomere unit is _____ mm
    a. 2   b. 2.5
    c. 3   d. 1.5
22. What is the minimum time required for a nerve impulse to travel through a reflex arc ?
    a. 20 ms   b. 15 ms
    c. 30 ms   d. 25 ms
23. Energy requirement to lower a load quickly than slowly is _____.
    a. Lesser   b. More
    c. Same   d. None of the above

24. Quadriceps femoris shows peak force at _____ range.
    a. Outer range
    b. Inner range
    c. Mid range
    d. Through out the range muscle force same
25. Delayed onset muscle soreness is most severe at
    a. 5-10 hours
    b. 10 – 30 hours
    c. 30 – 45 hours
    d. 45 – 60 hours
26. During clinical ligament stress test the stresses that produce strains within the _____ region is applied by an evaluator.
    a. Linear elastic
    b. Toe
    c. Plastic
    d. Yield stress
27. At slow speed injury the failure of ligament results in _____.
    a. Ligament disruption
    b. Avulsion
    c. Complete tear
    d. Mild tear
28. The ductility of dense collagen tissue increases when temperature increased up to
    a. 35^0 C
    b. 40^0 C
    c. 45^0 C
    d. 42^0 C
29. Repaired tendons which are immobilized for 3 weeks are _____ than tendons immediately after suture
    a. Stronger
    b. No
    c. Less stronger
    d. None of the above
30. A small carrying angle means there is a risk of _____.
    a. Inferior dislocation
    b. Posterior dislocation
    c. Superior dislocation
    d. Anterior dislocation
31. A pathologic increase of neck shaft angle is known as _____.
    a. Coxa vara
    b. Coxa valga
    c. Femoral anteversion
    d. Femoral retroversion

32. The hip joint congruence is best in _____ position.
    a. Flexion, adduction and internal rotation
    b. Flexion, abduction and external rotation
    c. Extension, abduction and external rotation
    d. Extension, adduction and internal rotation
33. Shear stress is more over the femoral neck in _____.
    a. Coxa vara
    b. Coxa valga
    c. Femoral anteversion
    d. Femoral retroversion
34. What is the major structure responsible for closed packed position of hip joint?
    a. Muscles
    b. Articular surfaces
    c. Ligaments
    d. Combinations of all three
35. Zone of weakness in femur is that _____.
    a. Where system trabeculae is relatively thin
    b. Blood supply is less
    c. muscle coverage is less
    d. Ligaments are slack
36. The trabecular system is weak in the spine _____.
    a. Anteriorly   b. Posteriorly
    c. Laterally   d. In the middle
37. The ratio of disc thickness and vertebral body weight is maximum in which spine
    a. Lumbar   b. Thoracic
    c. Sacral   d. Cervical
38. The range of abduction of shoulder is less when shoulder is _____.
    a. Externally rotated   b. Internally rotated
    c. In neutral   d. In flexion
39. Static stabilization of glenohumeral articular surface is provided by _____.
    a. Coracohumeral ligament
    b. Coraco clavicualr ligament
    c. Superior joint capsule
    d. Coraco humeral ligament and superior joint capsule

40. Which is the most important muscle to produce upwards rotation of the scapula?
   a. Serratus anterior   b. Trapezius
   c. Levator scapulae   d. Deltoid
41. Which muscle around the hip is analogous to deltoid?
   a. Gluteus maximus   b. Gluteus minimus
   c. Gluteus medius   d. Iliopsoas
42. Apart from hip abductors which other muscles in the hip joint contribute to stability in bilateral stance?
   a. Extensors   b. Adductors
   c. Rotators   d. Flexors
43. For a person who weighs 60 kg how much weight comes on midstance on the stance limb?
   a. 40 kg   b. 50 kg
   c. 30 kg   d. 55 kg
44. Joint reaction force can be reduced to a maximum in case of hip joint pathology, if the patient _____.
   a. Leans to the affected side
   b. Leans to the unaffected side
   c. Carries a walking stick on the same side of pathology
   d. Carries a stick on the opposite side
45. The chances of neck of femur fracture is more in _____.
   a. Coxa valga   b. Coxa vara
   c. Femoral anteversion d. Femoral retroversion
46. Compressive forces in normal walking on knee joint is _____.
   a. 2 – 3 times body weight
   b. Same as body weight
   c. 4 – 5 times body weight
   d. None of the above
47. 5^0 of genu varum increases the compressive force on medial meniscus to _____.
   a. 25 %   b. 50 %
   c. 75 %   d. 10 %
48. Extensor retinaculum in the knee joint is _____.
   a. A part of capsule
   b. A part of extensor mechanism
   c. A part of quadriceps tendon
   d. None

49. Which structure contribute to abnormal lateral force on patella?
    a. TFL   b. IT Band
    c. LCL   d. None of the above
50. In a flexed knee rotation in either direction stretches structure.
    a. PCL   b. ACL
    c. MCL   d. LCL
51. Which knee joint ligament helps in locking?
    a. ACL   b. PCL
    c. LCL   d. Posterior capsule
52. During knee extension in weight bearing position _____ continues to move till the end of extension.
    a. Lateral condyle of femur
    b. Medial condyle of femur
    c. Head of the femur
    d. Condyles of tibia
53. The axis of rotation lies in _____ during locking of knee.
    a. Medial condyle
    b. Intercondylar region
    c. Lateral condyle
    d. None of the above
54. The role of gastrocnemius at knee is _____.
    a. Static stabilizer
    b. Mobilizer for flexion
    c. Dynamic stabilizer
    d. Synergistic for knee flexion
55. Which muscle is not included in pes anserinus?
    a. Gracilis   b. Semimembranosus
    c. Semi tendinosus   d. Sartorius
56. Which two muscles act to prevent entrapment of menisci during knee motion?
    a. Semitendinosus and popliteus
    b. Semimembranosus and popliteus
    c. Sartoris and popliteus
    d. Gastrocnemius and popliteus

57. The resultant pull of quadriceps femoris in frontal plane is _____.
    a. 7 to 10 medially
    b. 15 to 20 laterally
    c. 10 to 15 medially
    d. 15 to 20 laterally
58. At which knee flexion angle the moment arm is maximum?
    a. 45
    b. 60
    c. 90
    d. 30
59. Force production capacity due to loss of patella is most evident at_____.
    a. Closed kinematic chain last stage of knee extension
    b. Open kinematic last stage of knee extension
    c. Closed kinematic last stage of knee extension with resistance
    d. Open kinematic last stage extension with resistance
60. Patellofemoral joint reaction force is maximum at _____.
    a. Knee extension force
    b. 15^0 knee flexion
    c. 60^0 knee flexion
    d. 100^0 knee flexion
61. In squatting the JRF in patellofemoral joint may reach _____.
    a. 10 times of body weight
    b. 8 times of body weight
    c. 5 times of body weight
    d. 2 times of body weight
62. An increased Q angle depicts _____.
    a. Excessive medial force
    b. Excessive lateral force
    c. Excessive quadriceps force
    d. All of the three
63. Which is the commonest ligament injury in ankle?
    a. Calcaneo fibular
    b. Anterior talofibular
    c. Posterior talofibular
    d. LCL
64. _____ joint can withstand the most compressive force.
    a. Facet joint
    b. Hip joint
    c. Knee joint
    d. Ankle joint

65. The primary contributor to the resistance to passive stretching is _____.
    a. Cross bridges of myosin filament
    b. Titin
    c. Thixotrophy of muscle
    d. Stiffness of tendon
66. During forward reach _____ use lumbar spine movement earlier.
    a. Males   b. Females
    c. Children   d. Male and female equal
67. When the knee is flexed the pelvis tilts anteriorly, lumbar extension increases at 80^0 of knee flexion and knee can be flexed up to 135^0. But if the pelvis is stabilized the knee flexion stops at 90^0. What may be the reason?
    a. Normal rectus femoris length
    b. Short rectus femoris
    c. Stiff and short rectus femoris
    d. Stiff but not short rectus femoris
68. For runners a reduction of impact peak load can be achieved by _____.
    a. Forefoot striking
    b. Using suitable running shoe.
    c. Reducing weight
    d. b and c   e. All of the above.
69. Which is not a fault in genu recurvatum?
    a. Bowing of tibia and fibula on sagital plane
    b. Displacement of femur anterior to the tibia
    c. Inferior position of patella
    d. Weakening of posterior cruciate ligament
70. Which is not included in kinesiopathology of patellofemoral dysfunction?
    a. Insufficient gluteus medius
    b. Insufficient performance of vastus medialis
    c. Insufficient performance of iliopsoas
    d. Insufficient performance of gluteus maximus
71. There may be a rotation of the lumbar spine when the paraspinal side to side difference is greater than _____.
    a. 1"   b. 1.5"
    c. 2"   d. 0.5"

72. When the spine becomes flat there is increased pressure on the _____.
    a. Facets   b. Ligaments
    c. Disc   d. Body
73. Low back pain patient _____ muscle is an important contributor to the symptoms
    a. Erector spine   b. Iliopsoas
    c. Obliques   d. Hip extensors
74. Which is not a major cause of low back pain?
    a. Abdominals not controlling rotation between spine and pelvis
    b. Abdominals not preventing anterior pelvic tilt
    c. Abdominals not supporting isometrically the trunk
    d. Abdominals not supporting the trunk with an eccentric contraction
75. A subtalar pronation will_____.
    a. Increase the angle
    b. Decrease the angle
    c. Q angle will be unchanged
    d. None
76. Which is not a cause of low back pain?
    a. Abdominals not controlling rotation between spine and pelvis.
    b. Abdominals not preventing anterior pelvic tilt.
    c. Abdominals not supporting isometrically the trunk.
    d. Abdominals not supporting the trunk with an eccentric contraction.
77. Which muscle is the little helper of latissimus dorsi?
    a. Teris minor   b. Teres major
    c. Posterior deltoid d. Subscapularis
78. Second class lever will always have a lever arm _____.
    a. Equal to 1   b. More than 1
    c. Less than 1   d. More than 2
79. In which accessory movement multiple points along one articular surface contact multiple points on another articular surface?
    a. Slide   b. Rotation
    c. Spin   d. Roll

80. In which condition muscle force production is more?
    a. Less velocity middle range
    b. More velocity middle range
    c. Less velocity outer range
    d. More velocity inner range
81. Following tissue stabilize Gleno humeral joint except____.
    a. Coraco humeral ligament
    b. Superior capsule of the glenohumeral joint
    c. Biceps brachi
    d. Rotator Cuff
82. Structure which may get impinged in impingement syndrome are the following except_____.
    a. Subacromial bursa
    b. Superior capsule of glenohumeral joint
    c. Long head of biceps
    d. Conoid ligament
83. The arthrokinematics of shoulder flexion is _____.
    a. Roll and slide along joints longitudinal diameter
    b. Roll and slide along transverse diameter
    c. Spin movement of articular surface
    d. A roll of the articulating surface
84. During complete shoulder abduction the clavicular movement is _____.
    a. Elevation and anterior rotation
    b. Elevation and posterior rotation
    c. Depression and posterior rotation
    d. Depression and posterior rotation
85. In pulled elbow syndrome there is dislocation of _____.
    a. Radiohumeral joint
    b. Radioulnar joint
    c. Humeroulnar joint
    d. All of the above
86. Which muscle has the most efficient working capacity among elbow flexors?
    a. Biceps brachi
    b. Brachialis
    c. Brachioradialis
    d. Almost same work done by all the muscles

87. In triceps paralysis which shoulder muscle can substitute for it?
    a. Anterior deltoid
    b. Posterior deltoid
    c. Supraspinatus
    d. Short head of biceps brachi
88. Kienbock disease affects_____.
    a. Scaphoid
    b. Lunate
    c. Trapezium
    d. Trapezoid
89. Which one among the following causes abnormal sitting?
    a. Knees in slightly higher horizontal plane than the hips
    b. Sitting as back as possible supporting the back.
    c. Shoulder in line with lumber spine
    d. Foot supported on floor
90. The structure which gives restraint in the maximum directions is _____.
    a. LCL
    b. ACL
    c. MCL
    d. PCL
91. While standing from sitting position pushing the hands on the arm rest
    a. Creates force in the direction of quadriceps force
    b. Reaction force is in opposite direction of quadriceps
    c. Reaction force in the direction of quadriceps
    d. Creates force to increase ankle fixation
92. Injury rate is higher in which of the following exercise training?
    a. Concentric
    b. Eccentric
    c. Plyometric
    d. In all of the above
93. The limitations of EMG is _____.
    a. Can not quantify muscle strength
    b. Satisfactory dynamic recording different
    c. Indication of muscle activity
    d. a and b
94. Rectification in EMG means _____.
    a. Filtering out high frequency segment
    b. Summing over time
    c. Taking absolute values of
    d. All of the above
95. Tendons fail at an _____ increase in length.
    a. 15 %
    b. 8 %
    c. 12 %
    d. 4 %

96. Centre of pressure means _____.
    a. Centre of gravity of foot
    b. Centre of gravity of the body
    c. Point of application of resultant GRF
    d. None of the above
97. The moment imposed on any body segment mostly depend upon _____.
    a. Moment created by gravity
    b. Moment created by GRF
    c. Acceleration of the centre of gravity
    d. b and c
98. When a person climbs stairs GRF moves upward and forward. The work done is _____.
    a. Force X upward distance
    b. Force X upward distance + force X horizontal distance
    c. Force (Upward + horizontal distance)
    d. None of the above
99. The sequence of motor unit recruitment is predetermined at_____.
    a. Brainstem level
    b. Basal ganglia level
    c. Cerebral level
    d. Spinal level
100. The force frequency relationship between tonic muscles is _____.
    a. Linear
    b. Ramp and plateau
    c. Curvilinear
    d. None of the above
101. The capability of a motor unit exerting force is measured from_____.
    a. The maximum twitch force
    b. Peak force of fused tetanus
    c. Both a and b
    d. Fused tetanus
102. Which motor units have greatest innervations and largest muscle fibres?
    b. Slow contracting
    b. Fatigue resistance
    c. Fast to fatigue
    d. Both b and c
103. Resting membrane potential depolarizes within_____.
    a. 21 days
    b. 2 days
    c. 2 hours
    d. 10 days

104. EMG can be quantified by measuring the amplitude of _____.
    a. Rectified EMG   b. Integrated EMG
    c. Filtered EMG   d. None of the above
105. The magnitude of EMG is related to _____.
    a. Concentric contraction
    b. Eccentric contraction
    c. Isometric contraction
    d. All the three
106. Effective lubrication of articular surfaces requires _____.
    a. Intermittent compression and distribution
    b. Adequate immobilization
    c. Congruent articular surface
    d. a and c
107. Hyaline cartilages are found in _____.
    a. IVD   b. Ears
    c. Epiglottis   d. Joints
108. Instability occurs at which degree sprain?
    a. 1 degree   b. 2 degree
    c. 3 degree   d. 2 and 3 degree
109. How many positions of joint equilibrium does stable joint have for functional loading?
    a. 1   b. 2
    c. 3   d. More than 3
110. Clinically change in stiffness of ligaments is detectable when there is rupture of _____.
    a. Minimum fibres
    b. 10 % fibres
    c. Vast majority of fibres
    d. Half of fibres
111. The density of bone is _____.
    a. % of mineralized tissue
    b. % of non mineralized tissue
    c. Mineralized tissue/total bone tissue volume
    d. Non mineralized tissue/total bone tissue volume
112. Which one of the following may cause abnormal sitting?
    a. Shoulder in line with lumbar spine
    b. Knees should be slightly higher horizontal plane than the hips

c. Should sit as back as possible supporting the back
  d. Foot supported on floor
113. In forward bending which is considered an impairment
  a. A final lumbar flexion of 25^0 to 30^0
  b. Lumbar flexion greater than 50 % of its total range
  c. A final lumbar flexion less than 30^0
  d. Lumbar flexion lesser than 50 % of its total range
114. While returning from trunk bending to standing posture which movement pattern is correct
  a. Lumbar extension followed by hip extension
  b. Lumbar extension followed by hip and spine extension
  c. Hip extension followed by spine extension
  d. Hip extension followed by hip and spine extension
115. Which may not be cause of disc injury
  a. Sitting at a desk rich for various office tools
  b. Golf
  c. Squash
  d. Tennis
116. The most important action of multifactor is
  a. Creating extension torque during lumbar extension
  b. Controlling anterior shear while forward bending
  c. Counteracting abdominals during rotation
  d. Exerting compressive force on lumbar spine
117. Obesity with large abdomen and buttock may be associated with
  a. Lumbar flexion syndrome
  b. Lumbar flexion rotation syndrome
  c. Lumbar extension syndrome
  d. Lumbar extension and rotation syndrome
118. In hip joint osteoarthritis the hypomobility is particularly for _____ movement.
  a. Extension   b. Flexion
  c. Abduction   d. Rotation
119. If the scapula is positioned more towards the c7 then there is shortening of _____ muscle.
  a. Trapezius
  b. Trapezius + levator scapulae and rhomboids
  c. Rhomboids and levator scapulae
  d. Trapezius and levator scapulae

120. The vertebral border of scapula is _____ inches away from midline
    a. 2"
    b. 3"
    c. 3.5"
    d. 2.5"
121. At completion of flexion vertebral border of scapula should be rotated_____.
    a. 30 degrees
    b. 45 degrees
    c. 50 degrees
    d. 60 degrees
122. Which is the key force couple in the scapular motion?
    a. Trapezius deltoid
    b. Deltoid serratus anterior
    c. Trapezius and serratus anterior
    d. Deltoid and rotator cuff
123. In zigzag deformity of the hand there is a gradual increase of moment arm of _____ muscle.
    a. FPL
    b. EPL
    c. APL
    d. FDS
124. Which muscle does not use pulley to define its moment arm in hand?
    a. FCR
    b. Extensors of wrist
    c. FCU
    d. a and b
125. Which muscle is the key extensor of the wrist because of its force production?
    a. ECRL
    b. ECRB
    c. ECU
    d. ED
126. Which muscle may not be an extensor of wrist when the forearm is pronated?
    a. ECRL
    b. Extensor digitorum
    c. ECRB
    d. ECU
127. Metacarpophalangeal joints of finger has _____ degrees of freedom.
    a. 1 degree
    b. 2 degree
    c. 3 degree
    d. More than 3
128. In functional position of hand which muscle length is kept at optimal length?
    a. Wrist extensor
    b. Wrist flexor
    c. Finger extensor
    d. Finger flexors

129. For meniscus injury there should be _____.
    a. Shear of compressed knee
    b. Torsion of compressed knee
    c. Shear and torsion of knee
    d. Torsion of extended knee
130. Inversion eversion component is more in_____.
    a. Ankle joint   b. Mild tarsal joint
    c. Subtalar joint   d. None of the above
131. Stance phase is _____ % of gait cycle
    a. 40 %   b. 50 %
    c. 60 %   d. 70 %
132. The most energy efficient gait is _____.
    a. Walking on usual walking habit
    b. Walking with a slower speed
    c. With brisk walking
    d. None of the above
133. Shin splint results due to _____.
    a. Flattened shortening of tibialis posterior
    b. Flattened medial longitudinal arch
    c. Loading phase is more demanding in sports
    d. All of the above.
134. The inability to control pronation by _____ results in tendonitis.
    a. Peroneus longus.
    b. Peroneus brevis
    c. Peroneus tertius.
    d. All of the above.
135. What type of exercises are best for improving bone strength?
    a. High impact exercises which generate GRF greater than twice body weight
    b. High impact exercise which generates GRF greater than body weight
    c. Low impact high repetition exercise
    d. Low impact long duration exercise.

136 Larger and possibly stronger bone is possible by _____.
   a. Exercising in adult hood.
   b. Exercising in child hood.
   c. Exercising after growth cease.
   d. Remaining physically active in childhood and adulthood

ANSWER SHEET OF BIOMECHANICS

1. c	2. b	3. b	4. c	5. d
6. a	7. a	8. a	9. b	10. b
11. a	12. c	13. b	14. c	15. b
16. c	17. c	18. a	19. c	20. a
21. b	22. c	23. a	24. c	25. d
26. b	27. b	28. b	29. b	30. c
31. b	32. b	33. a	34. c	35. a
36. a	37. d	38. b	39. d	40. b
41. b	42. b	43. b	44. d	45. b
46. a	47. b	48. a	49. b	50. b
51. b	52. b	53. c	54. c	55. a
56. b	57. a	58. b	59. d	60. d
61. b	62. b	63. b	64. d	65. b
66. a	67. d	68. e	69. d	70. d
71. d	72. c	73. b	74. d	75. a
76. d	77. b	78. b	79. d	80. a
81. c	82. d	83. c	84. b	85. b
86. b	87. a	88. b	89. a	90. c
91. c	92. c	93. d	94. c	95. b
96. c	97. b	98. a	99. d	100. b
101. b	102. c	103. c	104. b	105. c
106. d	107. d	108. c	109. a	110. c
111. c	112. b	113. c	114. d	115. d
116. b	117. c	118. b	119. b	120. b
121. d	122. c	123. a	124. c	125. b
126. d	127. b	128. d	129. b	130. c
131. c	132. c	133. d	134. a	135. a
136. b				

CHAPTER 7

Rehabilitation

1. Mental retardation is a condition of arrested or incomplete development of mind, characterized by IQ____.
   a. Less than 100
   b. Less than 90
   c. Less than 80
   d. Less than 70
2. Category I visual disability (40% impairment) is present when visual acuity is ____ with correction.
   a. 6/9 – 6/18 in better eye and 6/24 – 6/36 worse eye
   b. 6/18 – 6/36 in better eye and 6/6 to nil
   c. 6/40 – 6/60 in better eye and 3/60 to nil
   d. 3/60 – 1/60 in better eye and finger count at 1" distance to nil
3. Moderate hearing impairment (40 – 50%) is said to occur when the dB level is____.
   a. 26 – 40 dB
   b. 41 – 60 dB
   c. 61 – 70 dB
   d. 71 – 90 dB
4. Disability reflects at the ____ level.
   a. Organ
   b. Individual
   c. Society
   d. None of the above
5. Impairment is defined as____.
   a. Loss of psychological, physiological or anatomical structure of function in a human being
   b. Lack of ability to perform an activity considered to be normal for a human being
   c. Inability perform the family and social role
   d. None of the above

6. The persons with disability act, 1995 adopted the proclamation on ___ of people with disability.
   a. Full participation
   b. Equalization of opportunity
   c. Protection of rights
   d. All of the above
7. How many National institutes are there in India to deal with persons with disabilities?
   a. 3　　　　　　　　b. 4
   c. 6　　　　　　　　d. 7
8. Travel concession available for the orthopaedically disabled persons are___.
   a. 75% in 3T AC, 50% in 2T AC and 1st class in train along with one escort, 50% if % of disability is 40-49 and full if % of disability is 50 or more in bus and 50% air fare with aids and appliance free of charges.
   b. 50% in train, bus and air for the persons with disability and one escort
   c. 50% in train, bus and air for the persons with disability
   d. 50% in train and bus if % of disability is 40-49 and full if % of disability is 50 or more in bus along with one escort and 50% air fare with aids and appliance free of charges
9. Foot wear modification helps to_____.
   a. Modify weight transfer pattern by shifting load from sensitive to tolerance area
   b. Correct flexible deformity and accommodate rigid deformity
   c. Limit motion of painful, inflamed and unstable joints
   d. All of the above
10. Ankle plantar flexion and knee flexion occurs together to minimize upward displacement of CG during normal human locomotion. Cushion heel __
    a. Reduces the impact at heel strike
    b. Allows foot flat with limited plantar flexion
    c. Reduces the knee flexion
    d. All of the above

11. Medial heel wedge is recommended for the correction of ___.
    a. Hind foot pronation
    b. Equinus foot
    c. Hind foot supination
    d. CTEV
12. Thomas heel is given in case of ___.
    a. Equines foot   b. Cavus foot
    c. Flat foot   d. CTEV
13. Foot wear modification for calcaneal spurs is _____.
    a. Heel wedge   b. Gouged out heel
    c. Heel cuff   d. Soft heel padding
14. UCBL insert is indicated for ___.
    a. Equines foot   b. Cavus foot
    c. Flat foot   d. CTEV
15. Orthotic management for Perthe's disease is _____.
    a. KAFO
    b. HKAFO
    c. HKAFO with ischeal seat
    d. Hip abduction orthosis with trilateral socket and rocker bottom
16. _____ splint is prescribed for claw hand deformity.
    a. Cock-up   b. Knuckle bender
    c. Pan cake   d. Short opponens
17. _____ splint is prescribed for a case of median nerve injury.
    a. Cock-up   b. Knuckle bender
    c. Pan cake   d. Short opponens
18. _____ splint is prescribed for buttonaire deformity.
    a. Cock-up   b. Knuckle bender
    c. Gutter   d. Short opponens
19. Single bar AFO with medial T-strap is helpful in correcting ___ deformity.
    a. Equines foot   b. Cavus foot
    c. Pronated foot   d. CTEV
20. Orthotic management of CTEV includes _____.
    a. Dennis-brown splint
    b. Modified foot wear with medial stiff and straight border, lateral heel and sole raised without heel

c. AFO with lateral T-strap
   d. All of the above
21. In case of hip pathology walking stick is provided on the _____
   a. Same side   b. Opposite side
   c. Both the side   d. Any side
22. A person with left hip pain is found to have limb length shortening on the affected side,
   a. Foot wear compensation should be provided on the affected side.
   b. Foot wear compensation should be provided on the affected side with 1" deficit
   c. Foot wear compensation should be provided on the affected side with ½" deficit.
   d. No foot wear compensation should be provided.
23. Percentage of permanent physical impairment in case of unilateral AK amputee up to 1/3rd of thigh is _____
   a. 85%   b. 80%
   c. 75%   d. 70%
24. A person has got loss of limb ROM 16% and loss of muscle strength 8%. Percentage of permanent physical impairment is _____
   a. 22.6%   b. 24.0%
   c. 54.7%   d. 71.8%
25. In AK prosthesis the foot piece is positioned in _____
   a. Inset   b. Outset
   c. Neutral   d. None of the above
26. The foot rotation at heel strike in case of AK amputee is due to _____
   a. Hard plantar flexion bumper
   b. Misalignment of knee bolt
   c. Foot outset
   d. None of the above
27. _____ scheme provides financial assistance/loan to the persons with interest under self employment programme.
   a. PMRY   b. DRI Scheme
   c. NHFDC   d. SJSY

28. Lateral wedging is given to correct _____
    a. Genu valgus   b. Genu varum
    c. Flat foot   d. None of the above
29. Single lateral bar KAFO with T-strap is given for correction of _____
    a. Genu valgum   b. Genu recurvatum
    c. Genu varum   d. Knee flexion
30. Sling seat in a wheel chair can cause _____
    a. Slouched posture
    b. Hip adduction and internal rotation
    c. Wind swept deformity
    d. Thoracic scoliosis
31. What should be seat width in adult wheel chair?
    a. 18 – 20 inches   b. 16-18 inches
    c. 14 – 18 inches   d. 10-12 inches.
32. A patient's family wants to build a ramp to the entrance of home. The proper grade for the ramp should be _____
    a. 1" of ramp for every foot of rise in height.
    b. 1" of ramp for every 1" of rise in height
    c. 1" of ramp for every 2" of rise in height
    d. 1 foot of ramp for every inch of rise in height.
33. To perform a sliding board or shoulder depression transfer, the patient's wheel chair must have _____
    a. Detachable foot rest
    b. Detachable arms
    c. Anti-tip bars
    d. Brake handle extension
34. Sacral sitting in wheel chair may be due to ____.
    a. Hypotonia
    b. Limited active hip flexion
    c. Lap belt located high
    d. All of the above
35. Energy consumption in wheel chair depends upon _____
    a. Width of tire
    b. Width of caster
    c. Weight of the wheel chair
    d. All of the above

36. Amputation is a destructive surgery. It can be made constructive if comfortable and functional prosthesis can be fitted, which depend on___.
    a. Support by the socket
    b. Suspension system
    c. Alignment of various parts
    d. All of the above
37. The advantages of total contact socket _____.
    a. Prevents edema
    b. Comfortable as load are distributed over larger area of contact
    c. Increases sensory feedback, so better is the control over the prosthesis
    d. All of the above
38. Modular prosthesis is contraindicated for the following except___.
    a. Farmer   b. River bed area
    c. Very short stump   d. Very long stump
39. Prosthetic foot wear are classified as___.
    a. Articulated   b. Non-articulated
    c. Energy storing   d. All of the above
40. Jaipur prosthetic foot provides___.
    a. More freedom of motion
    b. Can be used without foot wear and appropriate for rural amputees
    c. Good cosmetic appearance
    d. All of the above
41. Jaipur foot may not be appropriate for BK amputees with ___.
    a. Long stump   b. Medium stump
    c. Short stump   d. Knee disarticulation
42. Salesian suspension is used in case of___
    a. Transtibial prosthesis
    b. Transfemoral prosthesis
    c. Symes prosthesis
    d. None of the above

43. Genu recurvatum gait in case of BK prosthesis is due to _____.
    a. Prosthetic foot inset
    b. Foot outset
    c. Anterior displacement of socket
    d. Posterior displacement of socket
44. Genu varum gait deviation during the mid stance phase in BK prosthetisis is due to _____.
    a. Excessive prosthetic foot inset
    b. Excessive prosthetic foot outset
    c. Anterior displacement of socket
    d. Posterior displacement of socket.
45. Excessive heel cushion results into ____ gait.
    a. Foot slap following heel strike
    b. Inadequate knee flexion
    c. Climbing on heel sensation
    d. All of the above
46. Transtibial prosthesis with thigh corset is indicated in case of the following except__.
    a. Ideal stump
    b. Mediolateral knee instability
    c. Genu recurvatum
    d. Very short stump
47. Socket with soft lining is provided in cases of____.
    a. Diabetes
    b. Leprosy
    c. Bony prominence in the stump
    d. All of the above
48. Shoe with filler is given for ____ amputees.
    a. partial foot   b. Syme's
    c. BK   d. AK
49. Foot rotation following prosthetic heel strike in AK amputee is due to _____.
    a. Soft PF bumper
    b. Knee bolt not properly aligned
    c. Hard PF bumper
    d. Prosthetic foot in plantar flexion

50. An AK amputee demonstrates lateral trunk bending towards the affected side and pelvic drop on the prosthetic side during stance phase. The possible causes may be ____.
    a. Weakness of hip abductors
    b. Inadequate socket adduction
    c. Distalolateral discomfort in the stump
    d. All of the above
51. An AK amputee demonstrates lateral trunk bending, which can be observed from the ____.
    a. Back during the prosthetic mid stance phase
    b. Side during the stance phase
    c. Front during the swing phase
    d. Back during the mid-swing phase
52. Which cervical orthosis acts as a reminder to prevent unwanted movements?
    a. Soft cervical collar
    b. Rigid cervical collar
    c. Semi rigid cervical collar
    d. Halo system
53. Which spinal brace is indicated for the scoliosis with apex below T6?
    a. Miami   b. Boston
    c. Milwakee   d. None of the above
54. William's brace is otherwise known as ____ orthosis.
    a. Lumbosacral flexion control
    b. Lumbosacral flexion-extension control
    c. Lumbosacral flexion-rotation control
    d. Lumbosacral extension lateral control
55. Which of the following spinal orthosis controls LS flexion-extension?
    a. Taylor   b. Knight
    c. Haris   d. Taylor-Knight
56. The posterior pelvic band of the spinal orthosis should lie____.
    a. Below PSIS
    b. Above inferior edge of sacrum
    c. Above inferior edge of sacrum and below PSIS
    d. Above PSIS and below GT

57. Under ADIP scheme, aids and appliances are provided free of cost to the persons with disability having total income per month _____.
    a. Upto Rs. 5,000/-   b. Upto Rs. 6,500/-
    c. Upto Rs. 8,000/-   d. Upto Rs. 10,000/-.
58. Clients are persons who _____.
    a. Are diagnosed with impairment
    b. Are diagnosed with functional limitation
    c. Seek physiotherapy service for promotion of health
    d. None of the above
59. Functional limitation in Nagi model is similar to _____ in ICIDH
    a. Impairment   b. Disability
    c. Handicap   d. None of the above
60. Disability in Nagi model is similar to _____ in ICIDH
    a. Impairment   b. Disability
    c. Disease   d. Handicap
61. In the illness model of WHO terminologies like body function, activity and participation are used from_____.
    a. 1998   b. 2000
    c. 2002   d. 2003
62. Once a patient gives his informed consent for research, then_____.
    a. He cannot withdraw consent
    b. Withdrawl is subject to principal researcher's wish
    c. He can withdraw concent at any time without prejudice
    d. Legal intervention is necessary for the patient to withdraw
63. Physical therapist intervene at the level of _____.
    a. Impairment   b. Functional limitation
    c. Disability   d. All of the above
64. Physical therapist can help in _____.
    a. Primary prevention   b. Secondary prevention
    c. Tertiary prevention d. All of the above
65. Which of the following does not come under Ethics?
    a. Professional collegiability
    b. Advocacy for the client
    c. Allocation of resource
    d. None of the above

66. Which of the following is not considered as consumer?
    a. A patient in a nursing home
    b. Apatient in a government hospital
    c. A patient in a private hospital
    d. A patient in a clinic
67. Appeal against an order of national consumer protection commission can be made to _____.
    a. High court
    b. Supreme court
    c. Central tribunal
    d. Non of the above
68. Where was the first PT education in INDIA started?
    a. KEM, Mumbai
    b. CMC, Vellore
    c. GMC, Chennai
    d. Anand
69. World Confederation of Physical Therapists was formed in ___.
    a. 1951   b. 1953
    c. 1062   d. 1064
70. How many countries have been registered by WCPT?
    a. 92   b. 96
    c. 156   d. 174
71. When was IAP registered by WCPT?
    a. 1951   b. 1953
    c. 1962   d. 1981
72. When was Indian association of Physiotherapists formed?
    a. 1951   b. 1953
    c. 1962   d. 1981
73. Which of the following is important for medicolegal point of view?
    a. Documentation
    b. Written informed consent
    c. Realization of responsibility
    d. All of the above
74. _____ award is given for the best school/institute performance during students' forum of the annual conference of the Indian association of Physiotherapists.
    a. Utkal branch gold medal

b. Alka verma
   c. C.P. Nair
   d. India-Medico
75. _____ award is given for the best graduate of the year during the students' forum of the annual conference of the Indian association of Physiotherapists.
   a. Utkal branch gold medal
   b. Alka verma
   c. C.P. Nair
   d. India-Medico

ANSWER SHEET OF REHABILITATION

1. d	2. b	3. b	4. b	5. a
6. d	7. b	8. a	9. d	10. d
11. a	12. c	13. b	14. c	15. d
16. b	17. d	18. c	19. c	20. d
21. b	22. c	23. a	24. a	25. a
26. a	27. a	28. b	29. a	30. b
31. b	32. d	33. b	34. d	35. d
36. d	37. d	38. c	39. d	40. d
41. a	42. b	43. d	44. a	45. d
46. a	47. d	48. a	49. c	50. d
51. a	52. a	53. b	54. d	55. b
56. c	57. b	58. c	59. b	60. d
61. c	62. c	63. d	64. d	65. d
66. b	67. b	68. a	69. a	70. a
71. c	72. b	73. d	74. b	75. a

CHAPTER 8

Physiotherapy in Surgical Conditions

1. Low back pain during pregnancy is due to_____.
   a. Increased load of the apophyseal joints more
   b. Decrease in IVF size
   c. Pressure of Lumbosacral plexus
   d. All the above
2. Increased thoracic kyphosis in the pregnancy is to_____.
   a. Compensate for thoracolumbar lordosis to gain the balance
   b. Hide the enlarged breasts
   c. All the above
3. Thoracic outlet syndrome in pregnancy is due to_____.
   a. Rounded shoulders which reduces the valet size
   b. Fluid retention
   c. Elevation of first rib
   d. All of the above
4. Swelling in lower limb during pregnancy is due to _____.
   a. Pressure over inferior vena cava by the gravid uterus
   b. Vasodilation by the increased circulatory progesterone
   c. Gravity
   d. All of the above

5. During pregnancy oestrogen level is increased 30 times, which _____.
   a. Relaxes various pelvic ligaments to accommodate the gravid uterus
   b. Vasodilatation
   c. Affect metabolism
   d. None of the above
6. During pregnancy body temperature _____.
   a. Increases by 0.5% over normal farenhite reading
   b. Remains unchanged
   c. Decreases by 0.5% over normal farenhite reading
   d. None
7. Increased frequency of micturation during pregnancy is due to _____.
   a. Dilatation of the ureter by the action of progesterone
   b. Compression of uterus by gravid uterus
   c. Elongated urethra
   d. All
8. During 3rd trimester one should lie in _____.
   a. Supine
   b. Side lying on left side
   c. Side lying in right side
   d. Crook lying
9. One must avoid lying _____ during late pregnancy.
   a. Supine
   b. Side lying on left
   c. Side lying on right
   d. None
10. Early fatigue during pregnancy is due to _____.
    a. Dilution anaemia
    b. Increase in body weight
    c. Decrease in metabolism
    d. All
11. Relaxation _____.
    a. Serves energy
    b. Reduces pain threshold
    c. Reduces HR, BP, RR etc.,
    d. All

12. Listening to music is a passive mental technique for relaxation. This procedure is known as _____.
    a. Attention focusing
    b. Distraction
    c. Dissociation
    d. Interference
13. Attention focusing is a mental interference technique for relaxation. It involves _____.
    a. A passive perceptual interference
    b. An active intentional and purposeful mental activity which focuses on another process.
    c. Concentrating attention upon a non painful characteristic of the event
    d. None
14. Pain during labour arises from _____.
    a. Stretching of the cervix.
    b. Pressure over sacral plexus
    c. Stretch and pressure over pelvic organs, ligaments and muscles
    d. All
15. Pelvic inflammatory disease as the inflammation of _____.
    a. Uterus   b. Cervix
    c. Ovary   d. Fallopian tube
16. Complication of salpingitis is _____.
    a. Sterility   b. Intestinal obstruction
    c. Peritonitis   d. All
17. Physiotherapy modality suitable for pelvic inflammatory. disease is _____.
    a. US   b. SWD
    c. IFT   d. LASER
18. Suitable position for delivery is _____.
    a. Supine lying
    b. Side lying
    c. ½ lying with hips and knees flexed
    d. Crook lying
19. Function of pelvic diaphragm is to _____.
    a. Hold the bladder base and neck in intra-abdominal pressure

b. Forms the external sphincter and constricts during increased intra abdominal pressure
c. Supports the pelvic disease
d. All
20. Laxity and weakness of pelvic floor muscles arise due to _____.
    a. Stretching and tearing of pelvic muscles during delivery
    b. Partial denervation of pudental and pelvic nerves
    c. Old age
    d. All of the above
21. Stress incontinence is characterized by _____.
    a. Overflow of urine
    b. Involuntary loss of urine
    c. Continuous flow of urine
    d. Urgency
22. Passage of urine more number of time is known as frequency. Normal frequency of urination is _____.
    a. 7 times during waking hour and 2 times during night
    b. 7 - 10 times during waking and 3 times during night
    c. 10 – 12 times during waking and once during night
    d. None
23. Functions of the pelvic diaphragm can be checked by asking the patient to _____.
    a. Weight lifting
    b. Jumping
    c. Stop midflow of urine
    d. All
24. Foetal movement can be felt at around _____.
    a. 12 weeks   b. 16 weeks
    c. 18 weeksd.   20 weeks
25. normal birth weight of the child is _____.
    a. 2800 gm   b. 3000 gm
    c. 3200 gm   d. 3400 gm
26. Which muscles require to be strengthened in pregnancy?
    a. Neck flexion, abdominals, hip extension, knee extension
    b. Neck extension, abdominals hip flexion, knee extensors

  c. Neck flexion, back extension, hip extension, knee flexion
  d. Neck extension, back extension, hip flexion, hamstrings
27. Which are the muscles require to be stretched in pregnancy?
  a. Upper neck extensors, Scapular protractors, Lower back extensors, hamstrings and TA
  b. Neck flexion, scapular retractors, abdominals, quadriceps and TA
  c. Neck extension, scapular protraction, back extension, hamstrings and TA
  d. Neck flexion, scapular protraction, abdominals, quadriceps and dorsiflexors.
28. Diastasis recti is tested in crock lying position by asking the subject to raise head and shoulder to touch the knees, while therapist palpitating the gap between the recti at the midline at different levels . It is considered significant when the gap is_____.
  a. More than 1 cm   b. More than 2 cm
  c. More than 3 cm   d. More than 4 cm
29. _____ incision is a muscle splitting incision.
  a. Paramedian   b. Mcburnies
  c. Cocher's   d. Infraumbilical transverse
30. _____ incision is a muscle retracting incision
  a. Paramedian   b. Mcburnies
  c. Cocher's   d. Infraumbilical transverse
31. _____ incision is used for gasterectomy
  a. Left upper paramedian
  b. Right upper paramedian
  c. Left subcostal
  d. Midline
32. Advantages of infraumbilical transverse incision include _____.
  a. It is covered by garment so preferred by the ladies for cosmetic point of view
  b. Moves with the respiratory movement so less painful
  c. All the above

33. The advantages of paramedian incision ____.
    a. No muscle cut, so no hernia
    b. No damage to the nerve or vessels
    c. Can be extended up and down
    d. All of the above
34. The disadvantages of cocher's incision _____.
    a. Muscle cut so chance of hernia
    b. Damage to the intercostals nerve 7th, 8th and 9th
    c. Giving rise to upper quadrant paralysis
    d. All of the above
35. Complication of radical mastectomy include_____.
    a. Oedema upper limb
    b. Loss of shoulder movement
    c. Balance problem
    d. Cosmesis and psychological problem
    e. All of the above
36. After abdominal surgery abnormal lung function persists up to_____.
    a. 1 week   b. 3 – 4 weeks
    c. 2 weeks   d. 4 weeks
37. The sign of DVT_____.
    a. Edema ankle and foot
    b. Pain and tenderness medial aspect of lower calf
    c. Positive Homan's sign
    d. All of the above
38. Skin from uniovular twin having common placenta is also accepted, which is called _____.
    a. Autograft   b. Isograft
    c. Homograft   d. Heterograft
39. Skin grafting fails because of _____.
    a. Movement of the graft
    b. Foreign material or any other substance under the graft
    c. Infection
    d. All of the above
40. It takes about _____ for the graft to establish its own blood flow.
    a. 3 – 4 days   b. 7 – 10 days
    c. 3 weeks   d. 6 weeks

41. Following skin graft the part must be left undisturbed and active movement can be started after _____.
    a. 3 - 4 days   b. 7 - 10 days
    c. 21 days   d. 6 weeks
42. Following skin graft the part must be left undisturbed and passive movement can be started after _____.
    a. 3 - 4 days   b. 7 - 10days
    c. 21 days   d. 6 weeks
43. Following skin grafting in the leg, patient must be _____ to avoid hemorrhage underneath the grafted skin by the increased hydrostatic pressure.
    a. Leg must be non-dependant for 10days
    b. Given standing and gait training in the hydrotherapy
    c. Made to stand with the elastocrepe bandage
    d. All of the above
44. Mostly burn occurs at the kitchen and_____ is most hazardous.
    a. Wick stove   b. Gas stove
    c. Pressure stove   d. All of the above.
45. Which of the following is the better way to extinguish fire?
    a. Wrapped blanket
    b. Pour water
    c. Roll the victim on the floor.
    d. Call fire brigade.
46. Surface area burn is calculated by rule of nine. How much surface palm of the hand include?
    a. 1   b. 5
    c. 7   d. 9
47. Heterotrophic bone formation occurs in deep and large burn, which is characterized by pain and gradual restriction of range of motion. The management of which is _____.
    a. Rest   b. Exercise
    c. Ultrasound   d. Surgical excision.
48. Physiotherapy following acute burn include _____.
    a. Positioning in anti contracture and elevation
    b. Changing the position at regular interval

c. Early active movements
d. All of the above.
49. Physiotherapy for hypertrophic scar is____.
   a. US				b. PWB
   c. DTFM			d. Pressure garment
50. Stretching of the transferred tendon can be performed after ___.
   a. 3 weeks
   b. 6 weeks
   c. Once the strength of thr transferred muscle become G4
   d. After 6 weeks provided the power is G3+

ANSWER SHEET OF PHYSIOTHERAPY IN SURGICAL CONDITIONS

1. d	2. c	3. d	4. d	5. a
6. a	7. d	8. c	9. a	10. d
11. d	12. b	13. b	14. d	15. d
16. d	17. b	18. c	19. d	20. d
21. b	22. a	23. c	24. d	25. d
26. a	27. a	28. b	29. b	30. a
31. a	32. c	33. d	34. d	35. d
36. c	37. d	38. b	39. d	40. a
41. a	42. b	43. d	44. c	45. b
46. a	47. a	48. d	49. d	50. d

CHAPTER 9

Alternative Medicine

1. Yoga is as old as_____.
   a. 2000 years   b. 3000 years
   c. 4000 years   d. 5000 years
2. _____ is said to be the greatest yogi (mahayogi).
   a. Pasupatinath   b. Patanjali
   c. Manu   d. Budha
3. Eight- fold yoga-path is laid by___.
   a. Pasupatinath   b. Patanjali
   c. Manu   d. Budha
4. The yogic cleansing practice to cleanse the respiratory tract is known as ____.
   a. Basti   b. Sasti
   c. Neti   d. Dhanti
5. The asana, which can be done after meals to improve digestion is____.
   a. Bhujangasana   b. Dhanurasana
   c. Trikonasana   d. Vajrasana
6. The asana that stimulates the Thyroid secretion is____.
   a. Sarvangasana   b. Uttana padasana
   c. Sasankasana   d. Tadasana
7. Toe touching in long sitting position is —.
   a. Pashchimottanasana   b. Vajrasana
   c. Dhanurasana   d. Bhujangasana

8. Ardha Matsyendrasana (Half-twist posture) is useful for stretching _____ muscle.
   a. Hamstrings
   b. Rectus Femoris
   c. Piriformis
   d. Gastro-soleus
9. Which Asana flexes the whole body?
   a. Pawan Muktasana
   b. Bhujangasana
   c. Dhanurasana
   d. Matsyasana
10. In close standing, interlace the fingers and stretch them up over head to stand on the toes is known as _____ asana.
    a. Pascimatanasana
    b. Ardha Cakrasana
    c. Tadasana
    d. Salabhasana
11. Suryanamaskar has got _____ steps.
    a. 6
    b. 10
    c. 12
    d. 18
12. Dhanurasana can be used to stretch the _____.
    a. Back extensors
    b. Abdominals
    c. Back extensors and hip extensors
    d. Abdominals and hip flexors
13. Paschimottanasana stretches bilateral
    a. Hamstring
    b. Quadriceps
    c. Abdominals
    d. Gastrosoleus
14. Trikonasana with its variation cause _____.
    a. Lateral flexion of spine
    b. Rotation of spine
    c. Flexion of spine
    d. Lateral flexion and rotation of spine
    e. Extension and rotation of spine
15. Which of the following asanas does not cause abdominal strengthening?
    a. Utthanapadasana
    b. Chakrapadasana
    c. Padasanchalasana
    d. Padanguli namana
16. Which one among the following asanas can strengthen the abdominals as well as stretch the erector spine?
    a. Suptaudarakarshanasana
    b. Suptapawanamuktasana
    c. Sputa vajrasana
    d. None of the following

17. Which one amon te following is not a relaxation asana.
    a. Shavasana   b. Advasana
    c. Matsya kridasana   d. Tadasana
18. Bhujangasana causes spinal _____.
    a. Flexion   b. Extension
    c. Rotation   d. Lateral flexion
19. Salabhasana needs strong _____.
    a. Abdominals
    b. Back extensors
    c. Back and hip extensors
    d. All extensor of lowerlimb
20. Which asana is contraindicated for prolapsed inter vertebral disc?
    a. Ardhasalabhasana
    b. Bhujangasana
    c. Sarala dhanurasana
    d. Sputa pawanamukta asana
21. Which asana is contra indicaterd for spondylolisthesis?
    a. Chakrapadasana
    b. Suptapawanamukta asana
    c. Jhulanalurhakanasan
    d. Dhanurasana
22. Flexion and extension of spine is done by_____.
    a. Vyagrasana   b. Vajrasana
    c. Paschimottasana   d. None of the above
23. External rotation in one side and internal rotation in other side shoulder is done by——— asana.
    a. Manibandhachakra   b. Gomukhasana
    c. Dwikonasana   d. Triyaka tadasana
24. In periarthritis shoulder which asana can be prescribed _____.
    a. Manibandhachakra   b. Gomukhasana
    c. Dwikonasana   d. None of the above
25. Accupuncture is as old as_____.
    a. 500 years   b. 1000 years
    c. 5000 years   d. 10,000 years
26. The mental activities are controlled by_____.
    a. Ren and Du   b. H and Liv
    c. K and Du   d. H and Du

27. The mental activities are controlled by _____.
    a. Lungs   b. Heart
    c. Kidneys   d. Stomach
28. Correct couple organs among the followings are ____.
    a. Heart and pericardium
    b. Heart and small intestine
    c. Stomach and small intestine
    d. Stomach and lungs
29. Each meridian has _____ Jing-wel points.
    a. 2   b. 4
    c. 6   d. 8
30. The best accupuncture point in the boby is _____.
    a. Du-14   b. Du-20
    c. St-36   d. P-3l
31. The best expectorant point is___.
    a. St 44   b. St 36
    c. Sp 10   d. Sp 6
32. For tonification, use————.
    a. Jing-wel point   b. Yuang source point
    c. Alarm point   d. Local point
33. Filiform needle is of _____ gauge.
    a. 16   b. 18
    c. 24   d. 30
34. Moxibustion is mainly given for————.
    a. Sedation   b. Tonification
    c. Localised treatment d. Aromapathy
35. GV 20 is the best _____ point.
    a. Haemostatic   b. Tonifying
    c. Sedative   d. Immune enhancing pint
36. Which of the following is false with regard to Yin?
    a. Slid organ   b. Male
    c. Negative   d. Inner side of the limb.
37. Yin is ____ in nature.
    a. Dark   b. Light
    c. Positive   d. None of the above
38. Which is not a traditional component of 5 elements?
    a. Air   b. Wood
    c. Metal   d. Earth

39. The following is not an indication for acupuncture
    a. Alopecia   b. Asthma
    c. Eczema   d. Diabetes
40. Ah shi points are
    a. Meridian points   b. Floating points
    c. Alarm points   d. Match points
41. Human body is made up of ___ natural elements.
    a. 3   b. 4
    c. 5   d. 7
42. Who is known as the father of naturopathy?
    a. Vincenz Priesnitz b. Adolf Just
    c. Mahatma Gandhi   d. Goutam Buddha
43. According to naturopathy the root cause of all diseases _____.
    a. Germs
    b. Batta, pitta and cough
    c. Accumulation of morbid matters in the body
    d. Sora, sika and syphilis
44. In naturopathy, to get well from the acute diseases the patient should be kept on___.
    a. Same diet as before
    b. Only on veg. diet
    c. Fasting on water or natural fluid
    d. None of the above
45. In naturopathy Enema is applied to cleanse the___.
    a. Respiratory tract b. Large colon
    c. Stomach   d. Nose
46. _____ is the emergency point.
    a. LI–4   b. K–1
    c. LU–1   d. GB–20
47. At what time maximum energy flow in heart meridian?
    a. 12 midnight   b. 6 AM
    c. 12 noon   d. 6 PM
48. In nature cure fast, rest and evacuation are the treatment formula for _____.
    a. Acute diseases   b. Sub acute diseases
    c. Chronic diseases   d. Fatal diseases
    e. All of the above

49. Mud has remedial effects.
    a. 1   b. 2
    c. 3   d. 4
50. The nature cure method applied in naturopathy to conserve energy from digestion and to eliminate morbid matters quickly is _____.
    a. Mud packs   b. Baths
    c. Fasting   d. Sun bathing

ANSWER SHEET OF ALTERNATIVE MEDICINE

1. d	2. a	3. b	4. c	5. d
6. a	7. a	8. c	9. a	10. c
11. c	12. d	13. a	14. d	15. d
16. b	17. d	18. b	19. c	20. d
21. d	22. a	23. b	24. b	25. a
26. d	27. b	28. b	29. b	30. b
31. a	32. b	33. d	34. b	35. c
36. b	37. a	38. a	39. d	40. b
41. c	42. a	43. c	44. c	45. b
46. d	47. c	48. a	49. d	50. c

CHAPTER 10

Biostatistics

1. When the range of scores and subjects is more than 20 how the data should be organized?
    a. Rank order
    b. Simple frequency
    c. Group frequency
    d. None of the above
2. A frequency polygon is a _____.
    a. Bar graph
    b. Line graph
    c. Histogram
    d. None of the above
3. In a normal curve the mean, median and mode are _____.
    a. Scattered
    b. In one line
    c. In mid line
    d. At one side of the curve
4. A platykurtic curve may result from _____.
    a. Wide range of scores with low frequencies in the mid range
    b. Limited range of scores with extreme scores on mid range
    c. Most scores fall on the mid range
    d. None of the above
5. In positively skewed curve _____.
    a. The tail is in the positive direction
    b. The hump is in the negative direction
    c. Both a and b
    d. Hump is at the positive direction and tail in the negative

6. A score in the 60th percentile means _____.
   a. 60% of the total score
   b. Equal to surpass 60% of raw score
   c. Both a and b
   d. None of them is appropriate
7. Ceiling effect is _____.
   a. Phenomena that describes highest score
   b. Phenomena that shows less improvement in percentile at upper end of scale
   c. More improvement of percentile at upper end of scale
   d. None of the above
8. For skewed data which measure of variability is useful.
   a. Percentile
   b. Range of the datas
   c. Interquartile range
   d. None of the above
9. The average of the squared deviation from the mean is _____.
   a. Standard deviation   b. Variance
   c. Interquartile range   d. None of the above
10. The square rootof variaqnce is _____.
    a. Standard deviation   b. Interquartile range
    c. Mode   d. Standard error
11. Is the formula for _____.
    a. Variance   b. Mode
    c. Standard deviation   d. Standard error
12. The most common measure of variability is _____.
    a. Variance   b. Standard deviation
    c. Standard error   d. All of them
13. What is the standard deviation if the data represent a population _____.
    a. Variance   b. Semiinterquartile range
    c. Standard error   d. Standard deviation
14. SEM can be calculated from sample _____.
    a. Mean and standard deviation
    b. Standard deviation and sample size
    c. Variance and sample size
    d. None of the above

15. Population mean is _____.
    a. Sample mean+/- 2 SEM
    b. Sample mean +/- 1 SD
    c. Sample mean +/- 1 SEM
    d. Sample mean +/- 2 SD
16. α is directly related to _____.
    a. Z value
    b. Standard deviation value
    c. Standard error value
    d. Number of subjects
17. α depicts probability of being _____.
    a. Correct   b. Incorrect
    c. Correct or incorrect
18. When Z^3mean is positive the data is _____.
    a. Skewed positive   b. Skewed negative
    c. Normal   d. Normal kurtosis
19. Kurtosis is relative _____.
    a. Symmetry of the data
    b. Peakedness of the data
    c. Normalcy of the data
    d. Representation of mean, median and mode
20. The narrow the effect size _____.
    a. Less number of subjects are studied
    b. Enough number of subjects are studied
    c. Narrow confidence interval
    d. None of the above
21. Mean + 1.96 SD covers _____.
    a. 68% of area   b. 76% of area
    c. 95% of area   d. 98% of area
22. Favorable outcomes out of total number of possible outcomes is _____.
    a. Probability   b. Confidence interval
    c. Size effect   d. Statistical power
23. Power is _____.
    a. 1 – a   b. b
    c. 1 - b   d. a
24. Incorrectly rejecting null is _____.
    a. Type I error   b. 1 – Type 1 error
    c. Type 2 error   d. 1 – Type 2 error

25. Comparison of two independent samples with normal distribution in ration scale can be done by which statistical test _____.
    a. paired t   b. unpaired t
    c. mann whitney U   d. wilcoxon signed rank
26. A pre and post normally distributed categorical data can be statistically tested by _____.
    a. paried t   b. unapired t
    c. wilcoxon rank test d. wilcoxon signed rank
27. Mann whitney U test is alternative to _____.
    a. Chisquare test   b. Independent t
    c. Dependent t   d. Pearson
28. Population divided into two or more groups according to common characteristics is _____ sampling.
    a. simple random   b. systematic
    c. stratified   d. non probability
29. When N is 1000 and n=50, selecting every 20th member from the list is _____.
    a. simple random sampling
    b. systematic random sampling
    c. stratified sampling
    d. quota sampling
30. Door to door survey which sampling is preferable_____.
    a. simple random   b. non probability
    c. systematic   d. cluster
31. A well designed trails should have a power of at least_____.
    a. 0.2   b. 0.7
    c. 0.8   d. 0.95
32. $n = Z^2 \times SD^2$
    Clinically expected difference is appropriate for _____.
    a. proportion studies
    b. prevalence studies
    c. mean is the parameter of study
    d. descriptive study
33. Correlation term is used for assessing relationship between _____.
    a. categorical variables
    b. continuous and categorical variables

c. Continuous variables
d. Data in ratio scale

34. The graphical representation to depict correlation is by _____.
    a. Histograms
    b. pi charts
    c. Scatter plot
    d. None of the above

35. Spearman's rank correlation used to assess _____.
    a. Two normally distributed continuous variable
    b. One ordinal and one continuous variable
    c. Continuous variables at least one of which is not normally distributed
    d. Agreement between two continuous variables

36. For quantitative data inter rater reliability can be tested by _____.
    a. Pearson's product moment
    b. Spearman's rank correlation co-efficient
    c. Intracrass correlation coefficient
    d. Kappa coefficient

37. Qualitative data intra rater variability can be measured by _____.
    a. r
    b. ρ
    c. z
    d. k

38. The value of correlation coefficient is always _____.
    a. 0.
    b. +/-1.
    c. >1.
    d. <1.

39. In simple regression the dependent variables should be put in
    a. X – axis.
    b. Y – axis.
    c. X or Y axis.
    d. Z – axis.

40. Kandall's rank correlation coefficient assess relation between _____.
    a. Two ordinary variables
    b. Two continuous variables
    c. One ordinary, one continuous variable
    d. a and c

ANSWER SHEET OF BIOSTATISTICS

1. c	2. b	3. c	4. a	5. c
6. b	7. b	8. c	9. b	10. a
11. c	12. b	13. c	14. b	15. c
16. a	17. b	18. a	19. b	20. b
21. c	22. a	23. c	24. a	25. b
26. c	27. c	28. c	29. b	30. d
31. c	32. c	33. c	34. c	35. c
36. c	37. d	38. b	39. b	40. d